CHOOSING HEALTH HIGH SCHOOL

STD AND HIV

Betty M. Hubbard, EdD, CHES

ETR Associates
Santa Cruz, California
1997

D1307453

ETR Associates (Education, Training and Research) is a nonprofit organization committed to fostering the health, well-being and cultural diversity of individuals, families, schools and communities. The publishing program of ETR Associates provides books and materials that empower young people and adults with the skills to make positive health choices. We invite health professionals to learn more about our high-quality publishing, training and research programs by contacting us at P.O. Box 1830, Santa Cruz, CA 95061-1830, (800) 321-4407.

Betty M. Hubbard, EdD, CHES, is a professor of health sciences at the University of Central Arkansas in Conway. She holds a BSE in biology, an MS in counseling, an MSE in health education and has taught biology, science and health education in grades K through 12. She received a Presidential Citation from the Association for the Advancement of Health Education and served as a member of the Joint Committee for National Health Education Standards. In addition to university teaching responsibilities, she coordinates teacher training, conducts research and serves as an author and consultant for health education curricula and videos.

Choosing Health High School
    Abstinence
    Body Image and Eating Disorders
    Communication and Self-Esteem
    Fitness and Health
    STD and HIV
    Sexuality and Relationships
    Tobacco, Alcohol and Drugs
    Violence and Injury

Series Editor: Kathleen Middleton, MS, CHES
Text design: Graphic Elements
Illustrations: Nina Paley

Printed in the United States of America

10 9 8 7 6 5 4 3 2 1
ISBN 1-56071-523-5

Title No. H685

Contents

Contents

CONTENTS

CONTENTS

CONTENTS

CONTENTS

Masters

ACKNOWLEDGMENTS

Choosing Health High School was made possible with the assistance of dedicated curriculum developers, teachers and health professionals. This program evolved from *Entering Adulthood*, the high school component of the *Contemporary Health Series*. The richness of this new program is demonstrated by the pool of talented professionals involved in both the original and the new versions.

Developers

Nancy Abbey
ETR Associates
Santa Cruz, California

Susan C. Giarratano, EdD, CHES
California State University, Long Beach
Long Beach, California

Susan J. Laing, MS, CHES
Department of Veterans Affairs Medical Center
Birmingham, Alabama

Clint E. Bruess, EdD, CHES
University of Alabama at Birmingham
Birmingham, Alabama

Betty M. Hubbard, EdD, CHES
University of Central Arkansas
Conway, Arkansas

Donna Lloyd-Kolkin, PhD
Health & Education Communication Consultants
New Hope, Pennsylvania

Dale W. Evans, HSD, CHES
California State University, Long Beach
Long Beach, California

Lisa K. Hunter, PhD
Health & Education Communication Consultants
Berkeley, California

Jeanie M. White, EdM, CHES
Education Consultant
Keizer, Oregon

Reviewers and Consultants

Brian Adams
Family Planning Council of Western Massachusetts
Northampton, Massachusetts

John Daniels
Golden Sierra High School
Garden Valley, California

Jon W. Hisgen, MS
Pewaukee Public Schools
Waukesha, Wisconsin

Janel Siebern Bartlett, MS, CHES
Dutchess County BOCES
Poughkeepsie, NY

Joyce V. Fetro, PhD, CHES
San Francisco Unified School District
San Francisco, California

Bob Kampa
Gilroy High School
Gilroy, California

Lori J. Bechtel, PhD
Pennsylvania State University, Altoona Campus
Altoona, Pennsylvania

Mark L. Giese, EdD, FACSM
Northeastern State University
Tahlequah, Oklahoma

Freya Klein Kaufmann, MS, CHES
New York Academy of Medicine
New York, New York

Judith M. Boswell, RN, MS, CHES
University of New Mexico
Albuquerque, New Mexico

Karen Hart, MS, CHES
San Francisco Unified School District
San Francisco, California

David M. Macrina, PhD
University of Alabama at Birmingham
Birmingham, Alabama

Marika Botha, PhD
Lewis and Clark State College
Lewiston, Idaho

Janet L. Henke
Old Court Middle School
Randallstown, Maryland

Linda D. McDaniel, MS
Van Buren Middle School
Van Buren, Arkansas

Wanda Bunting
Newark Unified School District
Newark, California

Russell G. Henke, MEd
Montgomery County Public Schools
Rockville, Maryland

Robert McDermott, PhD
University of South Florida
Tampa, Florida

ACKNOWLEDGMENTS

Carole McPherson, MA
Mentor Teacher Mission Hill Junior High School
Santa Cruz, California

Robert Mischell, MD
University of California, Berkeley
Berkeley, California

Donna Muto, MS
Mount Ararat School
Topsham, Maine

Priscilla Naworski, MS, CHES
California Department of Education
Healthy Kids Resource Center
Alameda County Office of Education
Alameda, California

Norma Riccobuono
La Paloma High School
Brentwood, California

Mary Rose-Colley, DEd, CHES
Lock Haven University
Lock Haven, Pennsylvania

Judith K. Scheer, MEd, EdS, CHES
Contra Costa County Office of Education
Walnut Creek, California

Michael A. Smith, MS, CHES
Long Beach Unified School District
Long Beach, California

Janet L. Sola, PhD
YWCA of the U.S.A.
New York, New York

Susan K. Telljohnn, HSD
University of Toledo
Toledo, Ohio

Donna J. Underwood, MS
Consulting Public Health Administrator
Champaign, Illinois

Peggy Woosley
Stuttgart Public Schools
Stuttgart, Arkansas

Dale Zevin, MA
Educational Consultant
Watsonville, California

PROGRAM OVERVIEW

COMPONENTS

PROGRAM GOAL

Students will acquire the necessary skills and information to make healthy choices.

Choosing Health High School consists of 8 Teacher/Student Resource books in critical topics appropriate for the high school health curriculum. *Think, Choose, Act Healthy, High School* provides creative activities to augment the basic program. There are also 13 *Health Facts* books that provide additional content information for teachers.

- **Teacher/Student Resource Books**—These 8 books address key health topics, content and issues for high school students. All teacher/student information, instructional process, assessment tools and student activity masters for the particular topic are included in each book.

- *Think, Choose, Act Healthy, High School*—This book provides 150 reproducible student activities that work hand in hand with the teacher/ student resource books. They will challenge students to think and make their own personal health choices.

- *Health Facts* **Books**—These reference books provide clear, concise background information to support the resource books.

PROGRAM OVERVIEW

COMPONENTS

Health Facts Books Correlation	
Resource Books	**Health Facts Books**
Abstinence	Abstinence Sexuality
Body Image and Eating Disorders	Nutrition and Body Image
Communication and Self-Esteem	Self-Esteem and Mental Health
Fitness and Health	Fitness
STD and HIV	STD HIV Disease
Sexuality and Relationships	Sexuality
Tobacco, Alcohol and Drugs	Drugs Tobacco
Violence and Injury	Violence Injury Prevention

Teaching Strategies

Each resource book is designed so you can easily find the instructional content, process and skills. You can spend more time on teaching and less on planning. Special tools are provided to help you challenge your students, reach out to their families and assess student success.

A wide variety of learning opportunities is provided in each book to increase interest and meet the needs of different kinds of learners. Many are interactive, encouraging students to help each other learn. The **31** teaching strategies can be divided into 4 categories based on educational purpose. They are Informational, Creative Expression, Sharing Ideas and Opinions and Developing Critical Thinking. Descriptions of the teaching strategies are found in the appendix.

Providing Key Information

Students need information before they can move to higher-level thinking. This program uses a variety of strategies to provide the information students need to take actions for health. Strategies include:

- anonymous question box
- current events
- demonstrations
- experiments
- games and puzzles
- guest speakers
- information gathering
- interviewing
- oral presentations

Encouraging Creative Expression

Creative expression provides the opportunity to integrate language arts, fine arts and personal experience into learning. It also allows students the opportunity to demonstrate their understanding in ways that are unique to them. Creative expression encourages students to capitalize on their strengths and their interests. Strategies include:

- artistic expression
- creative writing
- dramatic presentations
- roleplays

PROGRAM OVERVIEW

TEACHING STRATEGIES

Sharing Ideas, Feelings and Opinions

In the sensitive area of health education, providing a safe atmosphere in which to discuss a variety of opinions and feelings is essential. Discussion provides the opportunity to clarify misinformation and correct misconceptions. Strategies include:

- brainstorming
- class discussion
- clustering
- continuum voting
- dyad discussion
- family discussion
- forced field analysis
- journal writing
- panel discussion
- self-assessment
- small groups
- surveys and inventories

Developing Critical Thinking

Critical thinking skills are crucial if students are to adopt healthy behaviors. Healthy choices necessitate the ability to become independent thinkers, analyze problems and devise solutions in real-life situations. Strategies include:

- case studies
- cooperative learning groups
- debates
- factual writing
- media analysis
- personal contracts
- research

PROGRAM OVERVIEW

SKILLS INFUSION

Studies of high-risk children and adolescents show that certain characteristics are common to children who succeed in adverse situations. These children are called resilient. Evaluation of educational programs designed to build resiliency has shown that several elements are important for success. The most important is the inclusion of activities designed to build personal and social skills.

Throughout each resource book, students practice skills along with the content addressed in the activities. Activities that naturally infuse personal and social skills are identified.

- **Communication**—Students with effective communication skills are able to express thoughts and feelings, actively listen to others, and give clear verbal and nonverbal messages related to health or any other aspect of their lives.

- **Decision Making**—Students with effective decision-making skills are able to identify decision points, gather information, and analyze and evaluate alternatives before they take action. This skill is important to promote positive health choices.

- **Assertiveness**—Students with effective assertiveness skills are able to resist pressure and influence from peers, advertising or others that may be in conflict with healthy behavior. This skill involves the ability to negotiate in stressful situations and refuse unwanted influences.

- **Stress Management**—Students with effective stress-management skills are able to cope with stress as a normal part of life. They are able to identify situations and conditions that produce stress and adopt healthy coping behaviors.

- **Goal Setting**—Students with effective goal-setting skills are able to clarify goals based on their needs and interests. They are able to set realistic goals, identify the sub-steps to goals, take action and evaluate their progress. They are able to learn from mistakes and change goals as needed.

PROGRAM OVERVIEW

WORKING WITH FAMILIES AND COMMUNITIES

A few general principles can help you be most effective in teaching about health:

- Establish a rapport with your students, their families and your community.
- Prepare yourself so that you are comfortable with the content and instructional process required to teach about fitness and health successfully.
- Be aware of state laws and guidelines established by your school district that relate to health.
- Invite parents and other family members to attend a preview of the materials.

Family involvement improves student learning. Encourage family members and other volunteers to help you in the classroom as you teach these activities.

THE STD AND HIV RESOURCE BOOK

WHY TEACH ABOUT STD AND HIV?

Prevention is the key to protection against HIV and other STD. While some STDs can be treated and cured, the only way to protect against HIV is to prevent it. No successful vaccination or cure for HIV infection has yet been found.

This resource book of activities provides current information on STD, including HIV, in a framework designed to influence students' attitudes in a way that fosters healthy choices around sexual behavior.

STD, HIV and High School Students

The risk of contracting a sexually transmitted disease is very real for today's teenagers. Each year, millions of Americans are infected with a variety of STDs, including HIV. Experts estimate that approximately 1 in 8 teenagers gets an STD each year. Especially frightening is the spread of HIV among this population. At the end of 1991, more than 8,000 teenagers and young adults were diagnosed with AIDS. By 1992, the number of AIDS cases due to heterosexual transmission had increased by 65%.

Teens are particularly vulnerable to STD, including HIV infection, for many reasons. Developmentally, they are exploring their independence. They have a tendency to act impulsively, without considering long-term consequences of their actions. Many are experimenting with sex and with drugs and do not perceive themselves to be at risk through these activities. Also, conflicting feelings and embarrassment about sexuality may make communication about protection difficult.

Education about prevention of HIV and other STD through avoiding risky behaviors is the overall goal of these units. Behaviors addressed include sexual activity, drug use and activities in which blood is shared. Abstinence from such activities is the only 100% effective protection. The activities in this resource book promote sexual abstinence as the best means of protection for teens.

Teens who are sexually active must learn to protect themselves against HIV and other STD. Unit 6 covers the correct and consistent use of latex condoms. Students also investigate resources available to assist teens who are concerned about STD.

To prevent and protect against STD, including HIV, it is essential for students to gain effective communication, decision-making and assertive refusal skills. The activities included in this resource book emphasize skill practice.

The STD and HIV Resource Book

Why Teach About STD and HIV?

Background Information About STD and HIV

Instant Expert sections throughout this book give you all the information you need to teach each unit.

THE STD AND HIV RESOURCE BOOK

OBJECTIVES

Students Will Be Able to:

Unit 1: What Do You Know About STD?
- Describe STD, including HIV.

Unit 2: Pass It Around
- Categorize behaviors regarding the element of risk for contracting STD, including HIV.

Unit 3: Choosing Abstinence
- Analyze reasons for choosing abstinence.
- Demonstrate decision making that supports abstinent behavior.

Unit 4: Following Through on Abstinence
- Plan responses that reinforce the decision to be abstinent.
- Recognize nonverbal and verbal refusal skills.

Unit 5: Using Refusals
- Demonstrate refusals in roleplay situations.

Unit 6: Protection with a Capital C
- Demonstrate ways to talk to a partner about using condoms.
- Explain steps for male condom use.
- Survey products that provide protection from STD.

Unit 7: STD Symptoms, Consequences and Treatment
- Describe symptoms and consequences of STD.
- Identify and utilize sources for obtaining information, diagnosis and treatment of STD.

Unit 8: Understanding HIV
- Summarize essential information about HIV infection and prevention.

THE STD AND HIV RESOURCE BOOK

SAMPLE LETTER AND PERMISSION SLIP

Dear Family:

Your son or daughter will be involved in classes that focus on preventing sexually transmitted disease (STD), including HIV infection. Because these diseases are spread sexually, it is necessary to provide students with information about sexual behavior. The focus of these lessons will be prevention of infection. Abstinence will be promoted as the best choice for students; however, accurate information about other protection methods also will be provided.

Students will be practicing communication and decision-making skills throughout these lessons. Skills for refusing to become involved in risky behaviors will be emphasized.

You are invited to attend a preview of this course of study on

_____
(date, time)

at _____.
(place)

We will share the materials we will be using and hold an open discussion of STD and HIV prevention education.

We encourage you to talk to your son or daughter about this topic, sharing your knowledge and values. Please complete the permission slip at the end of this letter and have your son or daughter return it to school. Feel free to call if you have any questions.

Sincerely,

_____

- -

My son/daughter _____,
(name)

has permission to participate in the STD and HIV prevention education program.

I am interested in attending a preview night for parents and other family members.

Yes _____   No _____

_____ Date _____
(signature)

ANATOMY OF A UNIT

PREPARING TO TEACH

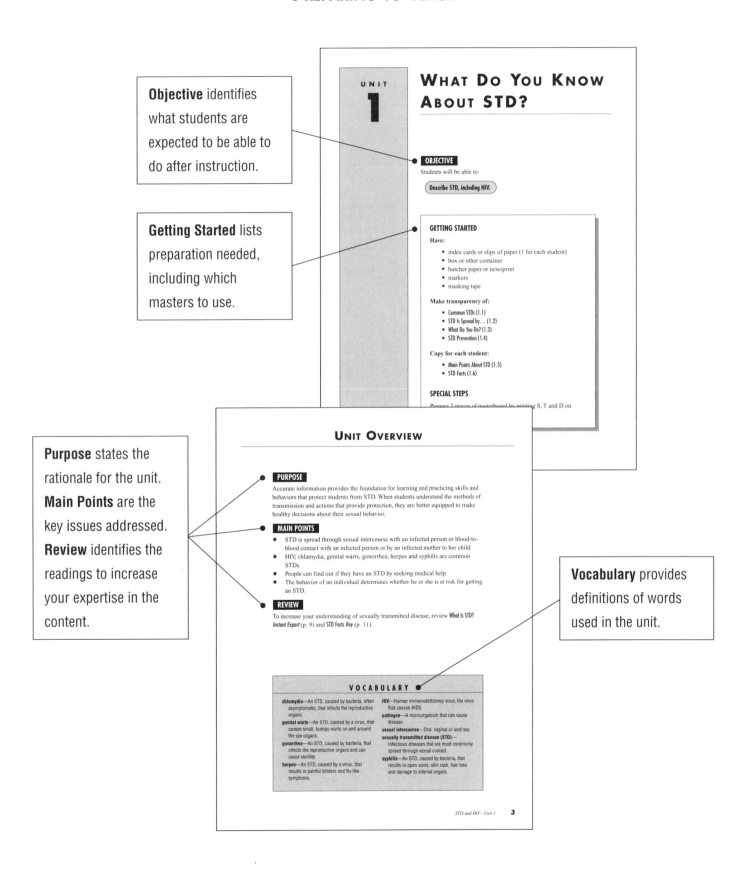

Objective identifies what students are expected to be able to do after instruction.

Getting Started lists preparation needed, including which masters to use.

Purpose states the rationale for the unit.
Main Points are the key issues addressed.
Review identifies the readings to increase your expertise in the content.

Vocabulary provides definitions of words used in the unit.

UNIT 1

WHAT DO YOU KNOW ABOUT STD?

OBJECTIVE

Students will be able to:

Describe STD, including HIV.

GETTING STARTED

Have:
- index cards or slips of paper (1 for each student)
- box or other container
- butcher paper or newsprint
- markers
- masking tape

Make transparency of:
- Common STDs (1.1)
- STD Is Spread by... (1.2)
- What Do You Do? (1.3)
- STD Prevention (1.4)

Copy for each student:
- Main Points About STD (1.5)
- STD Facts (1.6)

SPECIAL STEPS

Prepare 3 pieces of posterboard by printing S, T and D on

UNIT OVERVIEW

PURPOSE

Accurate information provides the foundation for learning and practicing skills and behaviors that protect students from STD. When students understand the methods of transmission and actions that provide protection, they are better equipped to make healthy decisions about their sexual behavior.

MAIN POINTS

* STD is spread through sexual intercourse with an infected person or blood-to-blood contact with an infected person or by an infected mother to her child.
* HIV, chlamydia, genital warts, gonorrhea, herpes and syphilis are common STDs.
* People can find out if they have an STD by seeking medical help.
* The behavior of an individual determines whether he or she is at risk for getting an STD.

REVIEW

To increase your understanding of sexually transmitted disease, review *What Is STD? Instant Expert* (p. 9) and *STD Facts Key* (p. 11).

VOCABULARY

chlamydia—An STD, caused by bacteria, often asymptomatic, that infects the reproductive organs.
genital warts—An STD, caused by a virus, that causes small, bumpy warts on and around the sex organs.
gonorrhea—An STD, caused by bacteria, that infects the reproductive organs and can cause sterility.
herpes—An STD, caused by a virus, that results in painful blisters and flu-like symptoms.

HIV—Human immunodeficiency virus; the virus that causes AIDS.
pathogen—A microorganism that can cause disease.
sexual intercourse—Oral, vaginal or anal sex.
sexually transmitted disease (STD)—Infectious diseases that are most commonly spread through sexual contact.
syphilis—An STD, caused by bacteria, that results in open sores, skin rash, hair loss and damage to internal organs.

STD and HIV—Unit 1   **3**

ANATOMY OF A UNIT

TEACHING THE ACTIVITIES

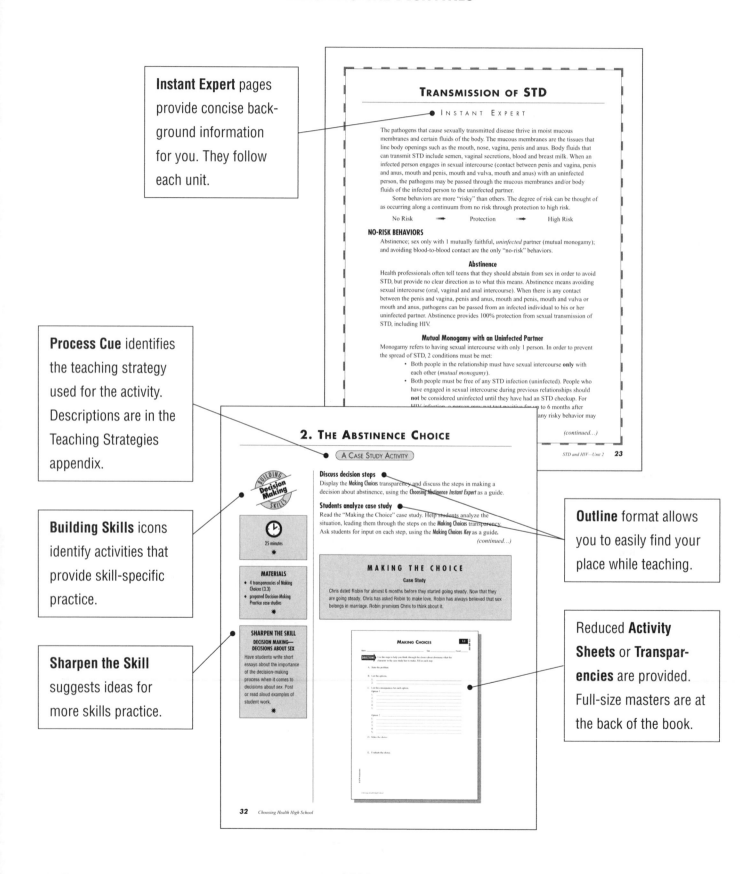

Instant Expert pages provide concise background information for you. They follow each unit.

Process Cue identifies the teaching strategy used for the activity. Descriptions are in the Teaching Strategies appendix.

Building Skills icons identify activities that provide skill-specific practice.

Sharpen the Skill suggests ideas for more skills practice.

Outline format allows you to easily find your place while teaching.

Reduced **Activity Sheets** or **Transparencies** are provided. Full-size masters are at the back of the book.

TRANSMISSION OF STD

● INSTANT EXPERT

The pathogens that cause sexually transmitted disease thrive in moist mucous membranes and certain fluids of the body. The mucous membranes are the tissues that line body openings such as the mouth, nose, vagina, penis and anus. Body fluids that can transmit STD include semen, vaginal secretions, blood and breast milk. When an infected person engages in sexual intercourse (contact between penis and vagina, penis and anus, mouth and penis, mouth and vulva, mouth and anus) with an uninfected person, the pathogens may be passed through the mucous membranes and/or body fluids of the infected person to the uninfected partner.

Some behaviors are more "risky" than others. The degree of risk can be thought of as occurring along a continuum from no risk through protection to high risk.

No Risk ⟶ Protection ⟶ High Risk

NO-RISK BEHAVIORS
Abstinence; sex only with 1 mutually faithful, *uninfected* partner (mutual monogamy); and avoiding blood-to-blood contact are the only "no-risk" behaviors.

Abstinence
Health professionals often tell teens that they should abstain from sex in order to avoid STD, but provide no clear direction as to what this means. Abstinence means avoiding sexual intercourse (oral, vaginal and anal intercourse). When there is any contact between the penis and vagina, penis and anus, mouth and penis, mouth and vulva or mouth and anus, pathogens can be passed from an infected individual to his or her uninfected partner. Abstinence provides 100% protection from sexual transmission of STD, including HIV.

Mutual Monogamy with an Uninfected Partner
Monogamy refers to having sexual intercourse with only 1 person. In order to prevent the spread of STD, 2 conditions must be met:
- Both people in the relationship must have sexual intercourse **only** with each other (*mutual monogamy*).
- Both people must be free of any STD infection (uninfected). People who have engaged in sexual intercourse during previous relationships should **not** be considered uninfected until they have had an STD checkup. For HIV infection, a person may not test positive for up to 6 months after [...] any risky behavior may

(continued...)

STD and HIV—Unit 2 **23**

2. THE ABSTINENCE CHOICE

(A CASE STUDY ACTIVITY)

Discuss decision steps ●
Display the *Making Choices* transparency and discuss the steps in making a decision about abstinence, using the *Choosing Abstinence Instant Expert* as a guide.

Students analyze case study ●
Read the "Making the Choice" case study. Help students analyze the situation, leading them through the steps on the *Making Choices* transparency. Ask students for input on each step, using the *Making Choices Key* as a guide.

(continued...)

BUILDING
**Decision
Making**
SKILLS

🕐
25 minutes
✳

MATERIALS
◆ 4 transparencies of Making Choices (3.3)
◆ prepared Decision-Making Practice case studies

SHARPEN THE SKILL
DECISION MAKING— DECISIONS ABOUT SEX
Have students write short essays about the importance of the decision-making process when it comes to decisions about sex. Post or read aloud examples of student work.
✳

MAKING THE CHOICE
Case Study
Chris dated Robin for almost 6 months before they started going steady. Now that they are going steady, Chris has asked Robin to make love. Robin has always believed that sex belongs in marriage. Robin promises Chris to think about it.

MAKING CHOICES

32 *Choosing Health High School*

ANATOMY OF A UNIT

SPECIAL FEATURES

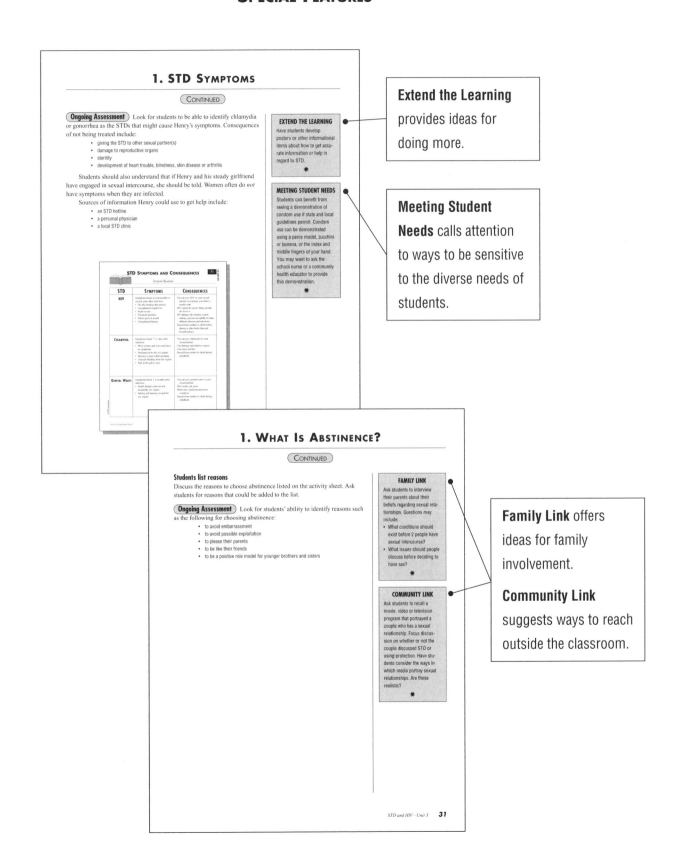

1. STD SYMPTOMS

CONTINUED

Ongoing Assessment Look for students to be able to identify chlamydia or gonorrhea as the STDs that might cause Henry's symptoms. Consequences of not being treated include:

- giving the STD to other sexual partner(s)
- damage to reproductive organs
- sterility
- development of heart trouble, blindness, skin disease or arthritis

Students should also understand that if Henry and his steady girlfriend have engaged in sexual intercourse, she should be told. Women often do *not* have symptoms when they are infected.

Sources of information Henry could use to get help include:

- an STD hotline
- a personal physician
- a local STD clinic

EXTEND THE LEARNING
Have students develop posters or other informational items about how to get accurate information or help in regard to STD.

MEETING STUDENT NEEDS
Students can benefit from seeing a demonstration of condom use if state and local guidelines permit. Condom use can be demonstrated using a penis model, zucchini or banana, or the index and middle fingers of your hand. You may want to ask the school nurse or a community health educator to provide this demonstration.

Extend the Learning provides ideas for doing more.

Meeting Student Needs calls attention to ways to be sensitive to the diverse needs of students.

1. WHAT IS ABSTINENCE?

CONTINUED

Students list reasons
Discuss the reasons to choose abstinence listed on the activity sheet. Ask students for reasons that could be added to the list.

Ongoing Assessment Look for students' ability to identify reasons such as the following for choosing abstinence:

- to avoid embarrassment
- to avoid possible exploitation
- to please their parents
- to be like their friends
- to be a positive role model for younger brothers and sisters

FAMILY LINK
Ask students to interview their parents about their beliefs regarding sexual relationships. Questions may include:
- What conditions should exist before 2 people have sexual intercourse?
- What issues should people discuss before deciding to have sex?

COMMUNITY LINK
Ask students to recall a movie, video or television program that portrayed a couple who has a sexual relationship. Focus discussion on whether or not the couple discussed STD or using protection. Have students consider the ways in which media portray sexual relationships. Are these realistic?

Family Link offers ideas for family involvement.

Community Link suggests ways to reach outside the classroom.

STD and HIV—Unit 3 **31**

ANATOMY OF A UNIT

EVALUATION FEATURES

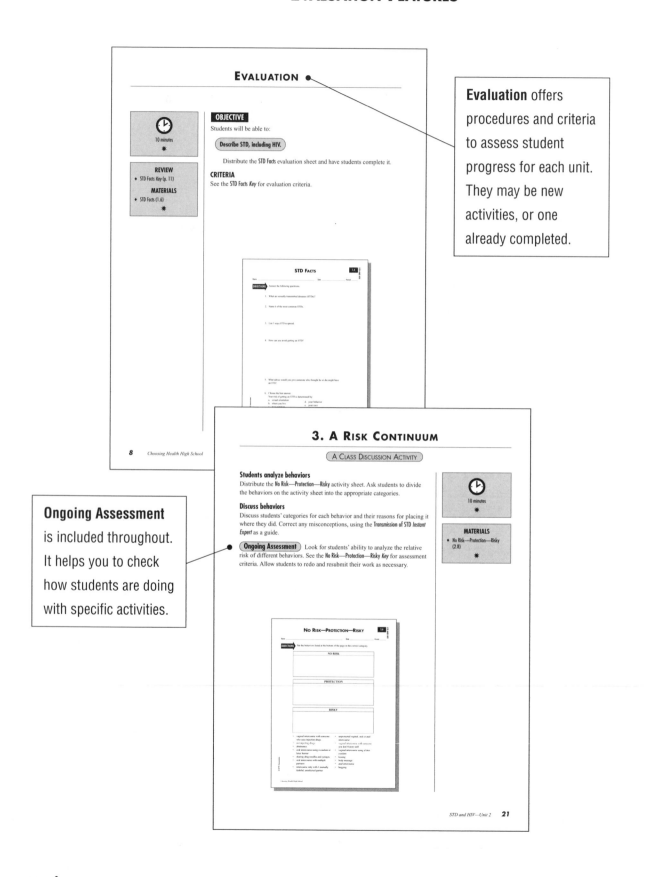

Evaluation offers procedures and criteria to assess student progress for each unit. They may be new activities, or one already completed.

Ongoing Assessment is included throughout. It helps you to check how students are doing with specific activities.

WHAT DO YOU KNOW ABOUT STD?

TIME

2 periods

ACTIVITIES

1. Trivial Pursuit

2. Questions About STD

3. Learning About STD

4. Answering Questions

WHAT DO YOU KNOW ABOUT STD?

OBJECTIVE

Students will be able to:

> Describe STD, including HIV.

GETTING STARTED

Have:

- index cards or slips of paper (1 for each student)
- box or other container
- butcher paper or newsprint
- markers
- masking tape

Make transparency of:

- Common STDs (1.1)
- STD Is Spread by... (1.2)
- What Do You Do? (1.3)
- STD Prevention (1.4)

Copy for each student:

- Main Points About STD (1.5)
- STD Facts (1.6)

SPECIAL STEPS

Prepare 3 pieces of posterboard by printing S, T and D on separate pieces. See Activity 1 (p. 4).

UNIT OVERVIEW

PURPOSE

Accurate information provides the foundation for learning and practicing skills and behaviors that protect students from STD. When students understand the methods of transmission and actions that provide protection, they are better equipped to make healthy decisions about their sexual behavior.

MAIN POINTS

✳ STD is spread through sexual intercourse with an infected person or blood-to-blood contact with an infected person or by an infected mother to her child.

✳ HIV, chlamydia, genital warts, gonorrhea, herpes and syphilis are common STDs.

✳ People can find out if they have an STD by seeking medical help.

✳ The behavior of an individual determines whether he or she is at risk for getting an STD.

REVIEW

To increase your understanding of sexually transmitted disease, review **What Is STD? Instant Expert** (p. 9) and **STD Facts Key** (p. 11).

VOCABULARY

chlamydia—An STD, caused by bacteria, often asymptomatic, that infects the reproductive organs.

genital warts—An STD, caused by a virus, that causes small, bumpy warts on and around the sex organs.

gonorrhea—An STD, caused by bacteria, that infects the reproductive organs and can cause sterility.

herpes—An STD, caused by a virus, that results in painful blisters and flu-like symptoms.

HIV—Human immunodeficiency virus; the virus that causes AIDS.

pathogen—A microorganism that can cause disease.

sexual intercourse—Oral, vaginal or anal sex.

sexually transmitted disease (STD)—Infectious diseases that are most commonly spread through sexual contact.

syphilis—An STD, caused by bacteria, that results in open sores, skin rash, hair loss and damage to internal organs.

1. TRIVIAL PURSUIT

5 minutes

MATERIALS

♦ posterboard pieces with the letters S, T and D

MEETING STUDENT NEEDS

Personal culture and experience will affect student views about STD. Habits, customs and beliefs about sexuality and sexual orientation are all part of this view. Be sensitive to the variety of beliefs and experiences that affect your students.

Pose question

Tell the class you have some *Trivial Pursuit* questions for them. The first question is, What disease are teens most likely to get? (Answer: the common cold.) Use the following clues to solicit responses until the question is answered:

Clue 1—This disease can be passed from parent to child, but is not inherited.
Clue 2—This disease may "change your voice."
Clue 3—This disease can make you sniff even when you're happy.
Clue 4—When you have this disease, your mouth is for breathing and your nose is for blowing.
Clue 5—The opposite of "hot."

Display letters

Have 3 students hold up the posterboard letters out of order in front of the class, for example, D T S. Explain to students that the letters are a clue about today's lesson. Ask the second *Trivial Pursuit* question: What is the second most common disease among teens? (Answer: STD.) Students can unscramble the letters to answer this question.

Discuss STD

Ask what the letters *STD* stand for. If necessary, explain that STD stands for sexually transmitted disease.

2. QUESTIONS ABOUT STD

Students write questions

Distribute index cards or slips of paper. Have students independently and anonymously write the question they would most like to have answered about STD.

Collect questions

Have students put the cards or slips of paper into a box.

Groups list questions

Divide students into groups of 5 and randomly distribute an equal number of questions from the box to each group. Give each group a piece of butcher paper or newsprint and a marker. Explain the group assignment:

- Read the questions but do not try to answer them.
- Eliminate any duplications and list the questions on butcher paper or newsprint.
- Add any questions generated in your group.
- Choose a reader to read your questions to the class.

Groups report

Have each group post its questions in the room while a group member reads them aloud. Eliminate any duplications.

Save the lists for use in Activity 4.

15 minutes

✳

MATERIALS

- index cards or slips of paper
- box or other container
- butcher paper or newsprint
- markers
- masking tape

MEETING STUDENT NEEDS

You may want to add a few important questions to the box to be sure they are covered in class discussion. You may also want to quickly preview students' questions before proceeding to the next step.

3. LEARNING ABOUT STD

A CLASS DISCUSSION ACTIVITY

15 minutes

MATERIALS

♦ transparency of Common STDs (1.1)

♦ transparency of STD Is Spread by... (1.2)

♦ transparency of What Do You Do? (1.3)

♦ transparency of STD Prevention (1.4)

♦ Main Points About STD (1.5)

COMMUNITY LINK

Invite a qualified speaker from a community organization such as the health department to present information on STD to students.

Discuss STD

Use the transparencies to emphasize the main points as you discuss STD. Refer to the **What Is STD?** *Instant Expert* as a guide.

Distribute the **Main Points About STD** activity sheet to each student as a follow-up to the discussion.

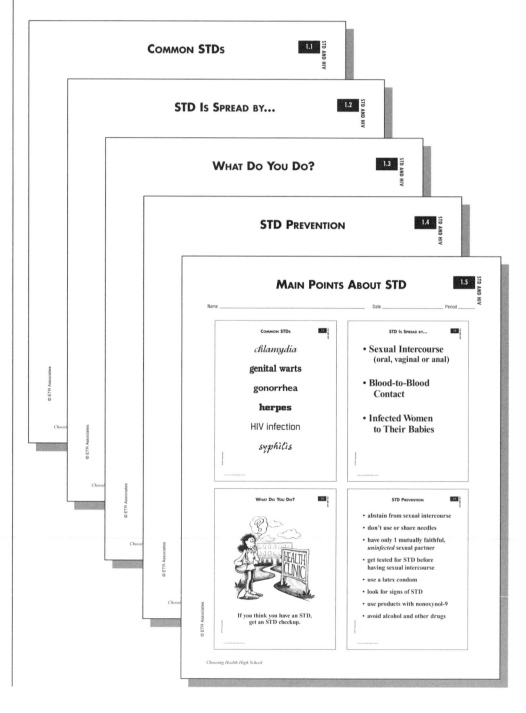

COMMON STDs — 1.1 — STD AND HIV

STD IS SPREAD BY... — 1.2 — STD AND HIV

WHAT DO YOU DO? — 1.3 — STD AND HIV

STD PREVENTION — 1.4 — STD AND HIV

MAIN POINTS ABOUT STD — 1.5 — STD AND HIV

Name _____ Date _____ Period _____

COMMON STDs

chlamydia

genital warts

gonorrhea

herpes

HIV infection

syphilis

STD Is Spread by...

• **Sexual Intercourse** (oral, vaginal or anal)

• **Blood-to-Blood Contact**

• **Infected Women to Their Babies**

WHAT DO YOU DO?

If you think you have an STD, get an STD checkup.

STD Prevention

• abstain from sexual intercourse

• don't use or share needles

• have only 1 mutually faithful, *uninfected* sexual partner

• get tested for STD before having sexual intercourse

• use a latex condom

• look for signs of STD

• use products with nonoxynol-9

• avoid alcohol and other drugs

4. ANSWERING QUESTIONS

Students answer questions

Have students return to their groups from Activity 2 and divide the questions equally among the groups. Explain the group assignment:

- Using the **Main Points About STD** activity sheet as a reference, discuss and attempt to answer the questions.
- Prepare to report your answers to the class.

Groups report

Have each group report their answers. Correct any misconceptions, using the **What Is STD?** *Instant Expert* as a guide.

20 minutes

MATERIALS

- lists of questions from Activity 2

EXTEND THE LEARNING

Ask students to bring in a newspaper or magazine article about STD. Tell them to underline the sections of the article that contain information discussed in class and to circle the sections of the article that contain information not discussed in class. Provide class time for students to share and discuss the information from the articles.

EVALUATION

10 minutes

REVIEW

♦ STD Facts *Key* (p. 11)

MATERIALS

♦ STD Facts (1.6)

OBJECTIVE

Students will be able to:

> **Describe STD, including HIV.**

Distribute the **STD Facts** evaluation sheet and have students complete it.

CRITERIA

See the **STD Facts** *Key* for evaluation criteria.

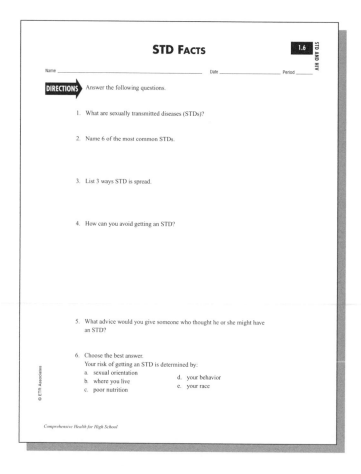

STD FACTS

				1.6

Name _____ Date _____ Period _____

DIRECTIONS Answer the following questions.

1. What are sexually transmitted diseases (STDs)?

2. Name 6 of the most common STDs.

3. List 3 ways STD is spread.

4. How can you avoid getting an STD?

5. What advice would you give someone who thought he or she might have an STD?

6. Choose the best answer.
   Your risk of getting an STD is determined by:
   a. sexual orientation
   b. where you live
   c. poor nutrition
   d. your behavior
   e. your race

© ETR Associates

Comprehensive Health for High School

WHAT IS STD?

Sexually transmitted disease, or STD, is the term used to identify a group of infectious diseases that are most commonly spread through sexual intercourse. STD is serious and can cause numerous health problems—physical, social and emotional.

STD used to be called VD, or venereal disease. The newer name reflects the diversity and large number of diseases that now comprise this group. Chlamydia, genital warts, gonorrhea, herpes, HIV and syphilis are common STDs.

Although each STD is a separate disease, all of the pathogens that cause STD are alike in that they thrive in the dark, warm, moist openings of the body (mouth, rectum, vagina and urethra). These pathogens may also be found in body fluids (blood, semen, vaginal secretions, breast milk, saliva and tears).

The incidence of STD is rising alarmingly, particularly among persons between ages 15 and 19. In fact, the only communicable disease a teenager is more likely to contract than an STD is the common cold.

Most STDs can be cured; some cannot. Sometimes a person can have an STD with no signs or symptoms. Other times the symptoms will disappear without treatment, but this does not mean the STD has been cured. Once infected with an STD, a person will remain infected until he or she gets medical treatment. For the incurable STDs (genital warts, herpes and HIV), a person remains infected even when provided with the best of medical care.

HOW DO PEOPLE GET STD?

People get STD through engaging in sexual intercourse with an infected partner. Sexual intercourse means oral, anal or vaginal intercourse. STD can also be passed from an infected mother to her child during pregnancy, birth or through breastfeeding. It can also be spread through contact with the blood of an infected person, such as by sharing needles and syringes for injecting drugs or sharing tattooing equipment or needles for piercing ears.

STDs, including HIV, are not transmitted through casual contact. An STD cannot be transmitted by sharing hairbrushes, shaking hands, using public toilets or hugging.

WHO GETS STD?

STDs, including HIV, affect people of both genders, from all age groups and from all socioeconomic levels, ethnic groups and regions of the world. Anyone who engages in behaviors that expose him or her to a pathogen that causes an STD is at risk for developing that sexually transmitted disease.

(continued...)

WHAT IS STD?

HOW CAN PEOPLE KNOW IF THEY HAVE AN STD?

People who have had oral, vaginal or anal intercourse or have shared a needle with someone who might have an STD should get an STD checkup. Only a qualified professional can administer the tests and prescribe treatment for an STD. You can't tell if a person has an STD by looking at them, so it is important for people to be tested if they think they have been exposed to an STD.

Many agencies and organizations provide information, diagnosis and treatment related to STD. Every effort is made to make sure that diagnosis and treatment is confidential and provided at minimal or no cost. In most states, minors can obtain information, diagnosis and treatment without the knowledge or consent of parents.

HOW CAN PEOPLE PREVENT STD?

People's behavior determines whether they are at risk for STD. Abstinence from sexual intercourse and refusing to share needles is the surest way to protect oneself from STD. Other things people can do to lower their chances of getting an STD include:

- Have only 1 mutually faithful, *uninfected* sexual partner—monogamy.
- Ask their partner to get tested *before* having sexual intercourse. STD tests are confidential, inexpensive and relatively painless.
- Use a latex condom or barrier.
- Look for any signs of a rash, a sore, redness or discharge from a partner's sexual organs. If there is anything unusual, **don't have sex!**
- Use products that contain nonoxynol-9. Birth control foams, creams, jellies, film and suppositories containing this product can kill some of the pathogens that cause STD.
- Avoid alcohol and other drugs. These can impair judgment about sexual decisions and behavior.

STD FACTS

KEY

DIRECTIONS Answer the following questions.

1. What are sexually transmitted diseases (STDs)?
   Diseases that are spread through sexual intercourse.

2. Name 6 of the most common STDs.
   - ***HIV***
   - ***chlamydia***
   - ***genital warts***
   - ***gonorrhea***
   - ***herpes***
   - ***syphilis***

3. List 3 ways STD is spread.
   - ***sexual intercourse with an infected person***
   - ***blood-to-blood contact with an infected person***
   - ***from an infected mother to her child during pregnancy or birth***

4. How can you avoid getting an STD?
   These are the only behaviors that are 100% effective:
   - ***Abstain from sexual intercourse.***
   - ***Refuse to share needles or other methods of blood-to-blood transmission.***
   - ***Mutual monogamy with an uninfected partner.***

   Other methods that decrease risk of STD include:
   - ***Using condoms and products containing nonoxynol-9.***
   - ***Avoiding alcohol and other drugs.***
   - ***Looking for rashes, sores and lumps on sexual partners.***

5. What advice would you give someone who thought he or she might have an STD?
   Get an STD checkup.

6. Choose the best answer.
   Your risk of getting an STD is determined by:
   a. sexual orientation
   b. where you live
   c. poor nutrition
   d. ***your behavior***
   e. your race

PASS IT AROUND

TIME

1–2 periods

ACTIVITIES

1. Pass It Around

2. Making Important Decisions

3. A Risk Continuum

PASS IT AROUND

OBJECTIVE

Students will be able to:

> Categorize behaviors regarding the element of risk for contracting STD, including HIV.

GETTING STARTED

Have:

- 2 latex gloves

Copy:

- Pass It Around—M1, M2, C, P?, A and I (2.1)–(2.6)

Copy for all but 6 students:

- Pass It Around (2.7)

Copy for each student:

- No Risk—Protection—Risky (2.8)

SPECIAL STEPS

Prepare materials for the Pass It Around Demonstration. See Activity 1 (p. 16).

UNIT OVERVIEW

PURPOSE

The activities in this unit present opportunities to explore feelings about STD infection. They illustrate behaviors that can eliminate, minimize or increase the risk of contracting an STD.

MAIN POINTS

✳ The pathogens that cause STD, including HIV, are most commonly transmitted through sexual intercourse.

✳ Certain behaviors can eliminate, reduce or increase the risk of getting an STD.

✳ "No-risk" behaviors include abstinence, not sharing needles or syringes, and only having sex with 1 mutually faithful, *uninfected* partner.

✳ "Protection" behaviors include protected vaginal intercourse (using a condom and a product containing nonoxynol-9) or protected oral intercourse (using a condom or a latex barrier).

✳ "Risky" behaviors include: sharing needles and syringes, anal intercourse, unprotected vaginal intercourse, unprotected oral intercourse, sexual intercourse with someone you don't know well, sexual intercourse while under the influence of drugs or alcohol, and sexual intercourse with multiple partners.

REVIEW

To increase your understanding of the role of behavior in the transmission of STD, review **Transmission of STD** *Instant Expert* (p. 23).

VOCABULARY

abstinence—Avoiding sexual intercourse.

latex barrier—A rectangular piece of latex used to cover the vulva during oral intercourse.

monogamy—Having only 1 sex partner.

mucous membranes—Tissues that line body openings.

no-risk behavior—Action that does not transmit STD.

protection behavior—Action that provides some protection against STD.

risky behavior—Action that may transmit STD.

vulva—External female genitalia.

1. PASS IT AROUND

30 minutes

MATERIALS

- Pass It Around—M1, M2, C, P?, A and I (2.1)–(2.6)
- 2 latex gloves
- Pass It Around (2.7)

Introduce demonstration

Explain to students that they are going to participate in an activity that will demonstrate how STD is spread and that a few of them have received special instructions. Distribute the **Pass It Around** activity sheet *without special instructions* to the remainder of the class. Explain the directions for the demonstration:

- Fold the activity sheet in half.
- When the teacher says, "Select a partner," select a person in the room, shake hands with the person and write her or his name on your activity sheet.
- Each time the teacher says, "Select a partner," select a new partner, shake hands and list the new partner's name on the activity sheet.
- Hold the instruction side of the sheet so no one else can see it.

Allow students to ask questions about the general directions before the activity begins.

Students perform demonstration

Give 5 opportunities for students to select a partner and shake hands. Allow time for students to write down their partners names between handshakes. After the fifth handshaking opportunity, have students sit down near their last partner.

Process demonstration

Tell students that there is a person who is "infected" with an STD in the group—the person with an "I" on his or her **Pass It Around** activity sheet. Have

(continued...)

PASS IT AROUND DEMONSTRATION

Prepare the **Pass It Around** activity sheets by copying and folding them. Before class begins, select 6 students to receive the **Pass It Around** activity sheets *with special instructions*—**M1, M2, C, P?, A** and **I**. Choose students who are not easily embarrassed.

Give the students with the **Pass It Around—C** and **Pass It Around—P?** activity sheets a latex glove. Allow all 6 students time to read the instructions on the activity sheets. Be sure they understand their special roles in this activity, but do not explain why they have special instructions at this time. Ask students to refrain from sharing their instructions until after the activity is completed.

---

1. PASS IT AROUND

students check their activity sheets and identify the person with the "I." Ask students questions such as the following:

- Is it really possible for an infected person to be unaware that he or she is infected? (Yes. It is possible for a person to have an STD and have no symptoms. For example, most people infected with HIV, the virus that causes AIDS, do not have any symptoms for many years.)
- What behaviors did the handshake stand for? (Sexual intercourse—vaginal, oral or anal intercourse.)

Discuss terms

Write the initial from each of the specialized activity sheets on the board along with the behavior for which it stood.

- A = abstinence (not participating in intimate sexual behavior)
- M1 and M2 = mutual monogamy
- C = condom use with nonoxynol-9
- P? = protection?
- I = infected

(continued…)

MEETING STUDENT NEEDS

Be sure students understand that the students with special characters on their activity sheets do **not** actually have those conditions. Emphasize that shaking hands is **not** a high-risk behavior but only stands for the high-risk behavior of unprotected sexual intercourse during the demonstration.

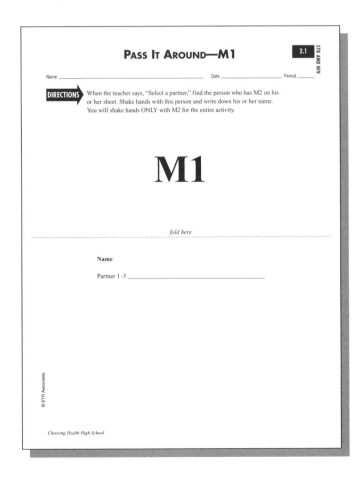

| PASS IT AROUND—M1 | 2.1 STD AND HIV |

Name _____ Date _____ Period _____

DIRECTIONS ▶ When the teacher says, "Select a partner," find the person who has M2 on his or her sheet. Shake hands with this person and write down his or her name. You will shake hands ONLY with M2 for the entire activity.

M1

fold here

Name

Partner 1–5 _____

© ETR Associates

Choosing Health High School

| PASS IT AROUND | 2.7 STD AND HIV |

Name _____ Date _____ Period _____

DIRECTIONS ▶ Shake hands with a new partner during each round and write down each partner's name.

fold here

Names

Partner 1 _____

Partner 2 _____

Partner 3 _____

Partner 4 _____

Partner 5 _____

© ETR Associates

Choosing Health High School

1. Pass It Around

Discuss the meaning of the terms *abstinence* and *mutual monogamy*, using the Transmission of STD *Instant Expert* as a guide.

Continue processing demonstration

Retrace each round of handshakes and have students check their activity sheets. The person in Round 1 who had unprotected "intercourse" (no glove) with the infected "I" individual became infected after that round. Have "I" and his or her first unprotected contact stand.

Check Round 2 for students who had unprotected contact with any of the students now standing and have them stand as well. Review each round, having all students who had unprotected contact with "infected" persons stand.

When a person with a glove (a student with Pass It Around—C or Pass It Around—P?) stands, explain that wearing the glove represented prevention by using a condom and spermicide containing nonoxynol-9. Ask students: What happened to the student with Pass It Around—P? in the last 3 rounds?

Discuss transmission risk

Discuss how the behaviors on each of the specialized activity sheets—Pass It Around—M1, M2, C, P?, A and I—relate to the risk of getting an STD, using the Transmission of STD *Instant Expert* as a guide.

Ask the students with Pass It Around—M1, Pass It Around—M2 and Pass It Around—A how they felt during the handshaking and during the discussion. How did the student with Pass It Around—I feel when he or she found out about being infected? Ask the class other questions such as the following:

- How did you feel about shaking hands with someone with a glove before you knew someone in the group was infected?
- Did your feelings change when you found out about the infected individual?

Ask students to think of some circumstances that would have changed the outcome of the demonstration. For example, what would have happened if:

- everyone had chosen 1 partner and had only shaken hands with that person?
- no one had shaken hands?
- everyone had worn gloves?
- 4 people in the class had been infected at the beginning of the activity?

2. MAKING IMPORTANT DECISIONS

A CASE STUDY ACTIVITY

Read case study

Read the "An Important Decision" case study to students.

Discuss case study

Discuss the case study with students, using questions such as the following:

- What are Jamie's options?
- Are any of these options "no risk"?
- Which provide protection?
- Which are "risky"?
- What would change in this situation if Jamie or Midori used injection drugs?
- Do you think most people are as open about discussing sexuality as Midori?
- How does withholding information about sexual behavior make decisions more difficult?
- Do you think Jamie would make a different decision if Midori had not told him about her past behavior?
- Why is abstinence the best choice for teens who want to avoid getting an STD, including HIV?

(continued...)

15 minutes

EXTEND THE LEARNING

Provide an opportunity for students to research the role of STD in history.

- What names were given to STD in the past?
- What treatments were used for STD?
- Which historical figures contracted STD?

AN IMPORTANT DECISION

Case Study

Midori moved to Atlanta during the middle of her junior year. She made many new friends and became involved in several school activities, including the student council. Midori was elected class president her senior year. Shortly after school started, Jamie asked her out and they began dating steadily.

About 3 months into the relationship, Midori began making sexual advances to Jamie. She made it clear to Jamie that she would like their relationship to include some intimate sexual behaviors. Wanting to be open in discussing sexuality, Midori told Jamie that she had had 2 sexual relationships before she moved to Atlanta.

Although very attracted to Midori, Jamie is a virgin and is not sure sexual intercourse is a good idea.

2. MAKING IMPORTANT DECISIONS

CONTINUED

FAMILY LINK

Have students interview their parents about teens and STD. Interview questions could include:

- How can teens protect themselves from STD?
- What could parents do to help their teens avoid STD?

Check students' comprehension

Look for students' ability to identify various options and the level of risk. Options might include:

- remain abstinent
- have unprotected oral, vaginal or anal intercourse
- have intercourse using a condom and a product containing nonoxynol-9
- ask Midori to get an STD checkup before having sexual intercourse

"No-risk" behaviors include:

- abstinence
- mutual monogamy (if Midori gets a checkup and is uninfected)

"Protection" behaviors include:

- vaginal intercourse with a condom and nonoxynol-9
- oral intercourse with a condom and a latex barrier (Point out that "protection" reduces the risk of getting an STD, but protection is not 100% effective.)

"Risky" behaviors include:

- unprotected oral and vaginal intercourse
- anal intercourse

Be sure students understand that if either Jamie or Midori used injection drugs, one or both of them could be infected. If he had ever injected drugs, Jamie would also need an STD checkup to make sure he was uninfected before having sexual intercourse with Midori. But if either of them continued to inject drugs or have other sexual relationships, the STD checkup would not be a good indicator of whether or not they were infected.

Students should also understand that it is difficult to make good decisions when you don't have all the facts and that some people are dishonest when discussing their sexual behavior.

3. A RISK CONTINUUM

Students analyze behaviors

Distribute the No Risk—Protection—Risky activity sheet. Ask students to divide the behaviors on the activity sheet into the appropriate categories.

Discuss behaviors

Discuss students' categories for each behavior and their reasons for placing it where they did. Correct any misconceptions, using the Transmission of STD *Instant Expert* as a guide.

Ongoing Assessment Look for students' ability to analyze the relative risk of different behaviors. See the No Risk—Protection—Risky *Key* for assessment criteria. Allow students to redo and resubmit their work as necessary.

10 minutes

MATERIALS

◆ No Risk—Protection—Risky (2.8)

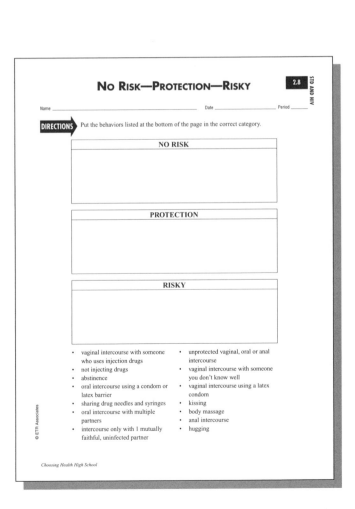

NO RISK—PROTECTION—RISKY | 2.8 | STD AND HIV

Name _____ Date _____ Period _____

DIRECTIONS Put the behaviors listed at the bottom of the page in the correct category.

NO RISK

PROTECTION

RISKY

- vaginal intercourse with someone who uses injection drugs
- not injecting drugs
- abstinence
- oral intercourse using a condom or latex barrier
- sharing drug needles and syringes
- oral intercourse with multiple partners
- intercourse only with 1 mutually faithful, uninfected partner

- unprotected vaginal, oral or anal intercourse
- vaginal intercourse with someone you don't know well
- vaginal intercourse using a latex condom
- kissing
- body massage
- anal intercourse
- hugging

© ETR Associates

Choosing Health High School

EVALUATION

REVIEW

- No Risk—Protection—Risky *Key* (p. 25)

MATERIALS

- completed No Risk—Protection—Risky (2.8), from Activity 3

OBJECTIVE

Students will be able to:

> **Categorize behaviors regarding the element of risk for contracting STD, including HIV.**

Assess students' work on the No Risk—Protection—Risky activity sheet for their ability to categorize behaviors according to the element of risk for STD.

CRITERIA

See the No Risk—Protection—Risky *Key* for evaluation criteria.

TRANSMISSION OF STD

The pathogens that cause sexually transmitted disease thrive in moist mucous membranes and certain fluids of the body. The mucous membranes are the tissues that line body openings such as the mouth, nose, vagina, penis and anus. Body fluids that can transmit STD include semen, vaginal secretions, blood and breast milk. When an infected person engages in sexual intercourse (contact between penis and vagina, penis and anus, mouth and penis, mouth and vulva, mouth and anus) with an uninfected person, the pathogens may be passed through the mucous membranes and/or body fluids of the infected person to the uninfected partner.

Some behaviors are more "risky" than others. The degree of risk can be thought of as occurring along a continuum from no risk through protection to high risk.

No Risk   ⟶   Protection   ⟶   High Risk

NO-RISK BEHAVIORS

Abstinence; sex only with 1 mutually faithful, *uninfected* partner (mutual monogamy); and avoiding blood-to-blood contact are the only "no-risk" behaviors.

Abstinence

Health professionals often tell teens that they should abstain from sex in order to avoid STD, but provide no clear direction as to what this means. Abstinence means avoiding sexual intercourse (oral, vaginal and anal intercourse). When there is any contact between the penis and vagina, penis and anus, mouth and penis, mouth and vulva or mouth and anus, pathogens can be passed from an infected individual to his or her uninfected partner. Abstinence provides 100% protection from sexual transmission of STD, including HIV.

Mutual Monogamy with an Uninfected Partner

Monogamy refers to having sexual intercourse with only 1 person. In order to prevent the spread of STD, 2 conditions must be met:

- Both people in the relationship must have sexual intercourse **only** with each other (*mutual monogamy*).
- Both people must be free of any STD infection (uninfected). People who have engaged in sexual intercourse during previous relationships should **not** be considered uninfected until they have had an STD checkup. For HIV infection, a person may not test positive for up to 6 months after being infected; therefore, a recheck 6 months after any risky behavior may be necessary.

(continued...)

TRANSMISSION OF STD

Avoiding Blood-to-Blood Contact

Blood-to-blood contact includes any situation in which the exchange of blood can occur. Such an exchange can take place through sharing needles or other equipment for injection drug use, sharing needles for ear piercing or tattooing, blood-brother/blood-sister rituals, blood transfusions or organ transplants.

To avoid risk of infection from blood-to-blood contact, never share needles or syringes for any purpose. In the United States, blood donated for transfusion is tested for STD before it is used and screening procedures are in place to prevent STD transmission through organ transplants. So the risk of contracting an STD through a medical procedure is very small.

PROTECTION BEHAVIORS

Protection behaviors can help prevent STD, but there is some risk that a condom or latex barrier might break or be used incorrectly. Using latex or polyurethane condoms and products with the spermicide nonoxynol-9 (found in contraceptive foams, creams, jellies, films and suppositories, and used with diaphragms as well as condoms) during vaginal intercourse and using condoms or latex barriers for oral intercourse (mouth and penis/vulva) provides some protection against the pathogens that cause STD. These behaviors are "protection" behaviors.

RISKY BEHAVIORS

Unprotected vaginal or oral intercourse, multiple sex partners, anal intercourse (protected and unprotected) and sharing needles and syringes are "risky" behaviors. Anal intercourse is a high-risk behavior because penetration of the rectum causes microscopic tears in the tissues, providing an ideal conduit for STD pathogens into the bloodstream.

Having sex while under the influence of alcohol or other drugs is also risky. When judgment is affected, people may not practice protection behaviors.

KEY

DIRECTIONS ➤ Put the behaviors listed at the bottom of the page in the correct category.

NO RISK
kissing
not injecting drugs
hugging
body massage
abstinence
intercourse only with 1 mutually faithful, uninfected partner

PROTECTION
oral intercourse using a condom or a latex barrier
vaginal intercourse using a latex condom

RISKY
sharing drug needles and syringes
unprotected vaginal, oral or anal intercourse
vaginal intercourse with someone who uses injection drugs
oral intercourse with multiple partners
vaginal intercourse with someone you don't know well
anal intercourse

- vaginal intercourse with someone who uses injection drugs
- not injecting drugs
- abstinence
- oral intercourse using a condom or latex barrier
- sharing drug needles and syringes
- oral intercourse with multiple partners
- intercourse only with 1 mutually faithful, uninfected partner
- unprotected vaginal, oral or anal intercourse
- vaginal intercourse with someone you don't know well
- vaginal intercourse using a latex condom
- kissing
- body massage
- anal intercourse
- hugging

CHOOSING ABSTINENCE

TIME

1–2 periods

ACTIVITIES

1. What Is Abstinence?
2. The Abstinence Choice
3. Making My Choice

CHOOSING ABSTINENCE

OBJECTIVES

Students will be able to:

> 1. Analyze reasons for choosing abstinence.

> 2. Demonstrate decision making that supports abstinent behavior.

GETTING STARTED

Copy for each student:

- About Abstinence (3.1)
- Reasons for Choosing Abstinence (3.2)
- Making My Choice (3.5)
- Abstinence Now (3.6)

Make 4 transparencies of:

- Making Choices (3.3)

Copy:

- Decision-Making Practice (3.4)

SPECIAL STEPS

Cut apart the case studies from the **Decision-Making Practice** teacher page. You may want to mount the case studies on card stock for reuse. See Activity 2 (p. 32).

UNIT OVERVIEW

PURPOSE

Activities in this unit provide students support for choosing abstinence as the best sexual behavior for teens. They encourage students to identify reasons for abstaining from intimate sexual behavior and steps to reinforce abstinent behaviors.

MAIN POINTS

* People choose abstinence for many reasons.
* Many teens choose abstinence.
* People can use decision-making steps to choose abstinence.

REVIEW

To increase your understanding of issues around abstinence, review **Choosing Abstinence Instant Expert** (p. 37) and **Making Choices Key** (p. 39).

VOCABULARY

abstinence—Avoiding sexual intercourse.

decision—The result of making up one's mind.

decision making—Making choices; using one's judgment.

1. WHAT IS ABSTINENCE?

25 minutes

MATERIALS

- About Abstinence (3.1)
- Reasons for Choosing Abstinence (3.2)

Students define abstinence

Have students write a definition of abstinence. Discuss their definitions and correct any misconceptions, using the **Choosing Abstinence** *Instant Expert* as a guide.

Students analyze choices

Distribute the **About Abstinence** activity sheet and ask students to complete it. Explain that this activity sheet is private and will not be shared with others in the class.

Discuss the situations on the activity sheet, using the **Choosing Abstinence** *Instant Expert* as a guide. Point out that abstinence was the choice made by Jessica, Marcus, Ashley and Jamal.

Students analyze reasons

Distribute the **Reasons for Choosing Abstinence** activity sheet and ask students to complete it.

(continued...)

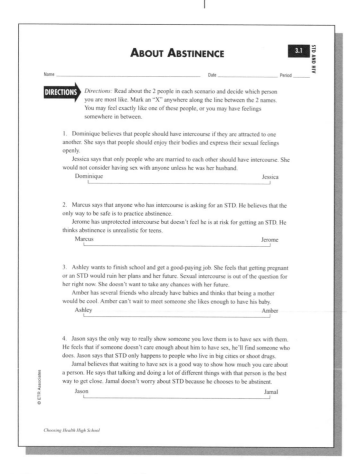

ABOUT ABSTINENCE   `3.1`   STD AND HIV

Name _____ Date _____ Period _____

DIRECTIONS ▶ *Directions:* Read about the 2 people in each scenario and decide which person you are most like. Mark an "X" anywhere along the line between the 2 names. You may feel exactly like one of these people, or you may have feelings somewhere in between.

1. Dominique believes that people should have intercourse if they are attracted to one another. She says that people should enjoy their bodies and express their sexual feelings openly.
   Jessica says that only people who are married to each other should have intercourse. She would not consider having sex with anyone unless he was her husband.
   Dominique _____ Jessica

2. Marcus says that anyone who has intercourse is asking for an STD. He believes that the only way to be safe is to practice abstinence.
   Jerome has unprotected intercourse but doesn't feel he is at risk for getting an STD. He thinks abstinence is unrealistic for teens.
   Marcus _____ Jerome

3. Ashley wants to finish school and get a good-paying job. She feels that getting pregnant or an STD would ruin her plans and her future. Sexual intercourse is out of the question for her right now. She doesn't want to take any chances with her future.
   Amber has several friends who already have babies and thinks that being a mother would be cool. Amber can't wait to meet someone she likes enough to have his baby.
   Ashley _____ Amber

4. Jason says the only way to really show someone you love them is to have sex with them. He feels that if someone doesn't care enough about him to have sex, he'll find someone who does. Jason says that STD only happens to people who live in big cities or shoot drugs.
   Jamal believes that waiting to have sex is a good way to show how much you care about a person. He says that talking and doing a lot of different things with that person is the best way to get close. Jamal doesn't worry about STD because he chooses to be abstinent.
   Jason _____ Jamal

© ETR Associates

Choosing Health High School

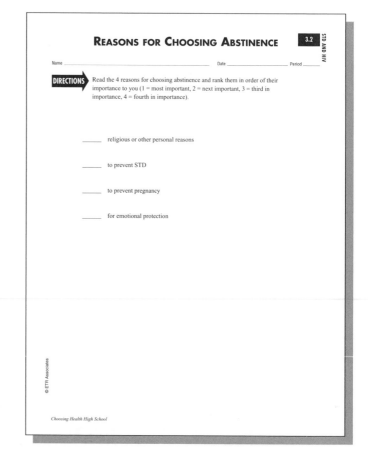

REASONS FOR CHOOSING ABSTINENCE   `3.2`   STD AND HIV

Name _____ Date _____ Period _____

DIRECTIONS ▶ Read the 4 reasons for choosing abstinence and rank them in order of their importance to you (1 = most important, 2 = next important, 3 = third in importance, 4 = fourth in importance).

_____ religious or other personal reasons

_____ to prevent STD

_____ to prevent pregnancy

_____ for emotional protection

© ETR Associates

Choosing Health High School

1. WHAT IS ABSTINENCE?

CONTINUED

Students list reasons

Discuss the reasons to choose abstinence listed on the activity sheet. Ask students for reasons that could be added to the list.

Ongoing Assessment Look for students' ability to identify reasons such as the following for choosing abstinence:

- to avoid embarrassment
- to avoid possible exploitation
- to please their parents
- to be like their friends
- to be a positive role model for younger brothers and sisters

---

FAMILY LINK

Ask students to interview their parents about their beliefs regarding sexual relationships. Questions may include:

- What conditions should exist before 2 people have sexual intercourse?
- What issues should people discuss before deciding to have sex?

2. THE ABSTINENCE CHOICE

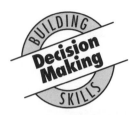

A CASE STUDY ACTIVITY

25 minutes

✳

MATERIALS

♦ 4 transparencies of Making Choices (3.3)

♦ prepared Decision-Making Practice case studies

✳

Discuss decision steps

Display the Making Choices transparency and discuss the steps in making a decision about abstinence, using the Choosing Abstinence *Instant Expert* as a guide.

Students analyze case study

Read the "Making the Choice" case study. Help students analyze the situation, leading them through the steps on the Making Choices transparency. Ask students for input on each step, using the Making Choices *Key* as a guide.

(continued...)

MAKING THE CHOICE

Case Study

Chris dated Robin for almost 6 months before they started going steady. Now that they are going steady, Chris has asked Robin to make love. Robin has always believed that sex belongs in marriage. Robin promises Chris to think about it.

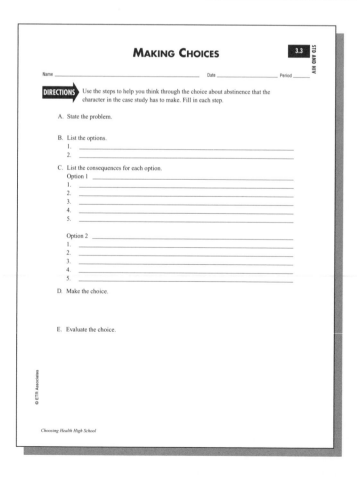

MAKING CHOICES   3.3   STD AND HIV

Name _____ Date _____ Period ____

DIRECTIONS ➤ Use the steps to help you think through the choice about abstinence that the character in the case study has to make. Fill in each step.

A. State the problem.

B. List the options.
1. _____
2. _____

C. List the consequences for each option.
Option 1
1. _____
2. _____
3. _____
4. _____
5. _____

Option 2 _____
1. _____
2. _____
3. _____
4. _____
5. _____

D. Make the choice.

E. Evaluate the choice.

© ETR Associates

Choosing Health High School

2. THE ABSTINENCE CHOICE

CONTINUED

Students practice making decisions

Divide the class into 3 small groups. Distribute a case study from the **Decision-Making Practice** teacher page to each group. Have each group record their steps on a **Making Choices** transparency as they work through the decision-making process for their case study.

Students share their work

Ask each group to read their case study, present their transparency and state their choice about abstinence.

Ongoing Assessment Assess students' ability to use the steps for decision making and to identify abstinence as the best choice for teens. If students choose sexual intercourse in Step D, acknowledge that there are strong pulls away from abstinence that will be considered later in the unit. Remind students that abstinence is the only 100% effective method for preventing pregnancy and sexual transmission of STD.

SHARPEN THE SKILL

DECISION MAKING—DECISIONS ABOUT SEX

Have students write short essays about the importance of the decision-making process when it comes to decisions about sex. Post or read aloud examples of student work.

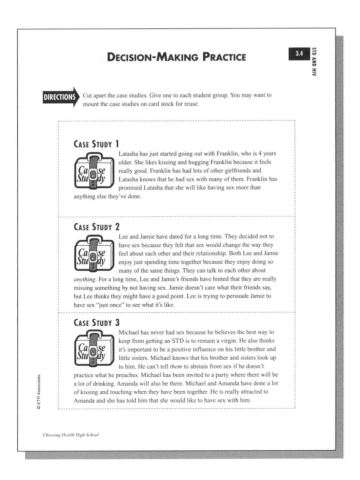

DECISION-MAKING PRACTICE　　3.4　STD AND HIV

DIRECTIONS Cut apart the case studies. Give one to each student group. You may want to mount the case studies on card stock for reuse.

CASE STUDY 1

Latasha has just started going out with Franklin, who is 4 years older. She likes kissing and hugging Franklin because it feels really good. Franklin has had lots of other girlfriends and Latasha knows that he had sex with many of them. Franklin has promised Latasha that she will like having sex more than anything else they've done.

CASE STUDY 2

Lee and Jamie have dated for a long time. They decided not to have sex because they felt that sex would change the way they feel about each other and their relationship. Both Lee and Jamie enjoy just spending time together because they enjoy doing so many of the same things. They can talk to each other about *anything*. For a long time, Lee and Jamie's friends have hinted that they are really missing something by not having sex. Jamie doesn't care what their friends say, but Lee thinks they might have a good point. Lee is trying to persuade Jamie to have sex "just once" to see what it's like.

CASE STUDY 3

Michael has never had sex because he believes the best way to keep from getting an STD is to remain a virgin. He also thinks it's important to be a positive influence on his little brother and little sisters. Michael knows that his brother and sisters look up to him. He can't tell *them* to abstain from sex if he doesn't practice what he preaches. Michael has been invited to a party where there will be a lot of drinking. Amanda will also be there. Michael and Amanda have done a lot of kissing and touching when they have been together. He is really attracted to Amanda and she has told him that she would like to have sex with him.

© ETR Associates

Choosing Health High School

3. MAKING MY CHOICE

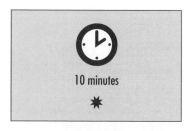

10 minutes

MATERIALS

◆ Making My Choice (3.5)

A PERSONAL CONTRACT ACTIVITY

Students make choices

Distribute the Making My Choice activity sheet. Explain that students can use the activity sheet to examine their own choices about sexual behavior. Emphasize that this activity sheet will be private, so students can be honest with themselves.

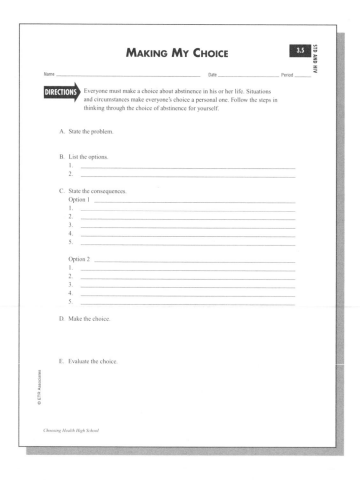

EVALUATION

OBJECTIVE 1

Students will be able to:

> **Analyze reasons for choosing abstinence.**

     Distribute the **Abstinence Now** evaluation sheet and have students complete it.

CRITERIA

See the **Reasons for Choosing Abstinence** activity sheet and **Choosing Abstinence** *Instant Expert* for evaluation criteria.

(continued...)

10 minutes

REVIEW

- Reasons for Choosing Abstinence (3.2)
- Choosing Abstinence *Instant Expert* (p. 37)

MATERIALS

- Abstinence Now (3.6)

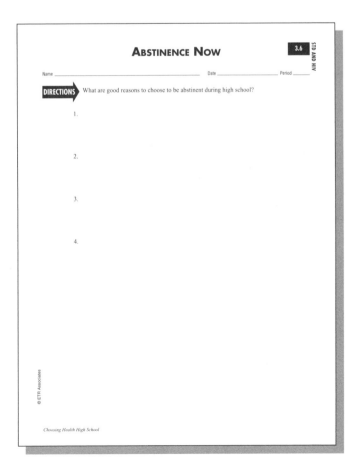

ABSTINENCE NOW   **3.6**   STD AND HIV

Name _____ Date _____ Period _____

DIRECTIONS What are good reasons to choose to be abstinent during high school?

1.

2.

3.

4.

© ETR Associates

Choosing Health High School

EVALUATION

CONTINUED

REVIEW

♦ Choosing Abstinence *Instant Expert* (p. 37)

MATERIALS

♦ completed Making Choices (3.3) transparencies, from Activity 2

OBJECTIVE 2

Students will be able to:

Demonstrate decision making that supports abstinent behavior.

Observe students' participation in the group decision making in Activity 2. Look for their ability to use the steps to reach a decision of abstinence.

CRITERIA

See the Making the Choice section of the **Choosing Abstinence** *Instant Expert* for evaluation criteria.

CHOOSING ABSTINENCE

Abstinence means avoiding sexual intercourse (including oral, vaginal and anal intercourse). Abstinence from sexual intercourse is 100% effective in preventing pregnancy and sexual transmission of sexually transmitted disease (STD).

REASONS FOR ABSTINENCE

There are many reasons for choosing abstinence. For many teens, the most important reason is a moral one. These teens believe that sexual intercourse belongs only in marriage for either religious or other personal reasons. Other teens feel that sexual intimacy belongs only in a serious relationship. They want commitment (a decision to continue the relationship) from the partner and they want to be committed to the partner.

Another obvious reason to abstain from sexual behavior is to avoid STD. People who choose to abstain from intercourse and from sharing needles and syringes are 100% protected from STD. Not having intercourse also provides 100% protection from pregnancy.

In addition to protecting teens from STD and pregnancy, abstinence also protects them emotionally. When people become close sexually, they open up a large part of themselves. They are likely to feel both intense happiness and intense pain. Sexual intercourse can be the most intimate way of sharing emotionally as well as physically. If a couple is not close enough to discuss all sorts of issues, including sex, pregnancy and STD, a decision to have intercourse may be premature.

EFFECTS OF CHOOSING ABSTINENCE

When people choose abstinence, the choice becomes part of their personal belief systems. People who have chosen abstinence and then engage in sexual intercourse may feel guilty and confused. Guilt and confusion occur when personal beliefs are not reflected in behavior.

For example, if Diego believes stealing is wrong, this is his personal belief. If Diego does not steal, his behavior is consistent with his personal beliefs. Positive feelings will result that will contribute to his sense of well-being. If Diego steals, his behavior is inconsistent with his beliefs. Feelings of confusion and guilt will follow.

(continued...)

CHOOSING ABSTINENCE

Some teens have the misconception that once people have intercourse, they are sexually active forever. This is not true. People move into sexual activity and back to abstinence for a variety of reasons. Married adults usually choose abstinence during separations from their partners (e.g., during business trips or illness). Divorced, widowed and never-married adults may practice abstinence for the same reasons as teens. Many teens who have had intercourse at one time or as part of a past relationship have chosen to return to abstinence.

MAKING THE CHOICE

As with all important decisions, sexual choices should be made when one has time to think carefully without being pressured. The best choices are made by going through a decision-making process. Steps in the process may include:

- Clarify the choices by specifically stating the problem.
- Consider the possible behaviors by listing the available options.
- Examine the possible outcomes by stating the consequences for each option.
- Make a choice based on these steps.
- Evaluate the choice to determine whether or not it was a good decision.

MAKING CHOICES

KEY

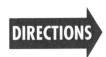 **DIRECTIONS** Use the steps to help you think through the choice about abstinence that the character in the case study has to make. Fill in each step.

A. State the problem.
   Should Robin have sex?

B. List the options.
   1. **Have sex now.**
   2. **Wait until marriage.**

C. List the consequences for each option.
   Option 1 **Have sex now.**
   1. **Robin will please Chris.**
   2. **Robin may feel guilty or disappointed.**
   3. **A pregnancy could occur.**
   4. **Robin might get an STD.**
   5. **Their parents might find out.**

   Option 2 **Wait until marriage.**
   1. **Marriage will be more special.**
   2. **Robin will feel good about the decision.**
   3. **Chris may feel angry or disappointed.**
   4. **Robin won't have to worry about STD.**
   5. **They won't have to worry about pregnancy.**

D. Make the choice.
   Answers may vary. Choices are not made based on the length of the list of positive or negative consequences, but rather on the individual's willingness to accept the perceived consequences.

E. Evaluate the choice.
   People evaluate their choices based on the consequences. If Robin chooses not to have sex right now, the decision can always be reevaluated later. If Robin chose to have sex and was unhappy with the consequences, Robin could make a different decision in the future, either with Chris or in future relationships. Unfortunately, however, a decision to have sex can have serious, irreversible consequences, such as pregnancy, STD or emotional upheaval.

FOLLOWING THROUGH ON ABSTINENCE

TIME

1–2 periods

ACTIVITIES

1. *Caution* Situations

2. Handling *Caution* Situations

3. *Danger* Situations

4. Convincing Refusals

FOLLOWING THROUGH ON ABSTINENCE

OBJECTIVES

Students will be able to:

> 1. Plan responses that reinforce the decision to be abstinent.

> 2. Recognize nonverbal and verbal refusal skills.

GETTING STARTED

Make transparency of:

- *Caution* Situations (4.1)
- *Danger* Situations (4.3)
- Refusals (4.4)

Copy 1 for each group:

- Handling *Caution* Situations (4.2)

Copy:

- How About a Date?—Unconvincing Version *Roleplay* (4.5), 2 copies
- How About a Date?—Convincing Version *Roleplay* (4.6), 2 copies

Copy for each student:

- Just This Once (4.7)

UNIT OVERVIEW

PURPOSE

Building on the decision to be abstinent in Unit 3, this unit focuses on situations that may lead to sexual intercourse. When students are able to identify these situations, they are better equipped to avoid the circumstances that may undermine their decision to be abstinent.

MAIN POINTS

* *Caution* and *danger* situations may threaten a person's decision to be abstinent.
* Teens can handle *caution* and *danger* situations.
* Nonverbal and verbal skills are a part of convincing refusals.
* Refusals can be used to remain abstinent.

REVIEW

To increase your understanding of *caution* and *danger* situations and refusals, review Following Through on Abstinence *Instant Expert* (p. 51).

VOCABULARY

body language—Forms of nonverbal communication that are clues to a person's thoughts and feelings.

caution situation—A circumstance that signals the approach of a *danger* situation.

danger situation—A circumstance that may lead to sexual intercourse unless immediate action is taken.

refusal—Saying no.

refusal skills—Ways to say no clearly and effectively while maintaining a relationship.

relationship building—Letting another person know one values the relationship.

1. CAUTION SITUATIONS

A CLASS DISCUSSION ACTIVITY

15 minutes

MATERIALS

♦ transparency of *Caution* Situations (4.1)

Discuss support for abstinence

Discuss ways to follow through on the choice to be abstinent, using the Following Through on Abstinence *Instant Expert* as a guide.

Students identify *caution* situations

Display the *Caution* Situations transparency and ask students to identify additional situations that would signal a "warning." Ask students to discuss ways they can respond to *caution* situations that follow through on their choice to be abstinent.

CAUTION SITUATIONS

- **Planning ways to be alone with a partner.**

- **Thinking about touching a partner.**

- **Planning to get and use alcohol or other drugs to relax.**

- **Dressing in a sexy way.**

© ETR Associates

Choosing Health High School

2. HANDLING *CAUTION* SITUATIONS

Triads respond to *caution* situations

Divide the class into groups of 3 and distribute a Handling *Caution* Situations activity sheet to each triad. Have students discuss and record responses that enable them to remain abstinent.

Triads share responses

Provide an opportunity for volunteers to share their groups' situations and responses.

Ongoing Assessment Look for students' ability to identify circumstances that could be categorized as *caution* situations and to develop responses that avoid or diffuse the situation. Students should demonstrate planning ahead to avoid being in a *danger* situation. See Following Through on Abstinence *Instant Expert* for specific criteria.

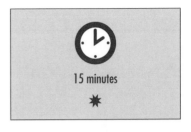

15 minutes

MATERIALS

♦ Handling *Caution* Situations (4.2)

MEETING STUDENT NEEDS

Remind students that, because we are all individuals, some approaches will feel more personally comfortable than others.

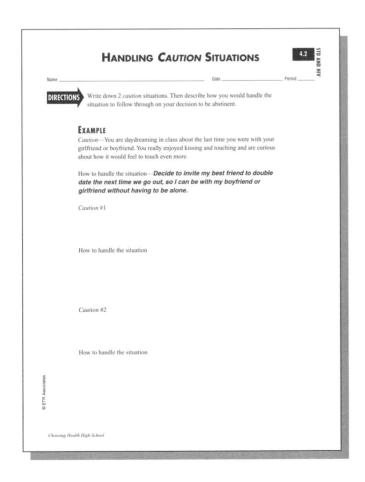

HANDLING *CAUTION* SITUATIONS   4.2   STD AND HIV

Name _____   Date _____   Period _____

DIRECTIONS Write down 2 *caution* situations. Then describe how you would handle the situation to follow through on your decision to be abstinent.

EXAMPLE

Caution—You are daydreaming in class about the last time you were with your girlfriend or boyfriend. You really enjoyed kissing and touching and are curious about how it would feel to touch even more.

How to handle the situation—**Decide to invite my best friend to double date the next time we go out, so I can be with my boyfriend or girlfriend without having to be alone.**

Caution #1

How to handle the situation

Caution #2

How to handle the situation

© ETR Associates

Choosing Health High School

3. DANGER SITUATIONS

A BRAINSTORMING ACTIVITY

10 minutes

MATERIALS

◆ transparency of *Danger Situations* (4.3)

◆ transparency of Refusals (4.4)

✸

Brainstorm *danger* situations

Display the *Danger* Situations transparency and ask students to brainstorm other situations that would be classified as *danger* situations. List student responses.

Discuss ways to handle *danger* situations

Discuss handling *danger* situations through the use of refusals. Use the Refusals transparency to acquaint students with the characteristics of a convincing refusal.

DANGER SITUATIONS `4.3` STD AND HIV

- **Touching each other in more ways.**

- **Getting sexually excited.**

- **Removing clothing.**

- **Lying down together.**

© ETR Associates

Choosing Health High School

REFUSALS   `4.4` STD AND HIV

1. **Send a nonverbal no (stand tall, firm expression, serious tone of voice).**

2. **Use the word *no*.**

3. **Repeat the no (as often as needed).**

4. **Suggest an alternate activity (something else to do).**

5. **Build the relationship (let other person know you value the relationship).**

© ETR Associates

Choosing Health High School

---

4. CONVINCING REFUSALS

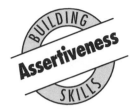

A ROLEPLAY ACTIVITY

Roleplay ineffective refusals

Ask 2 student volunteers to read the roleplays. Begin with How About a Date?—Unconvincing Version. Read the Background section to set the stage. Then have the volunteers perform the roleplay.

Discuss roleplay

Ask students to identify what Alicia did or did not do that made her refusal unconvincing.

Be sure the following points are made:

- Alicia never said *no.*
- She didn't repeat *no.*
- She wasn't clear and left Victor thinking she would go out with him.

(continued...)

20 minutes

MATERIALS

- How About a Date?—Unconvincing Version *Roleplay* (4.5)
- How About a Date?—Convincing Version *Roleplay* (4.6)

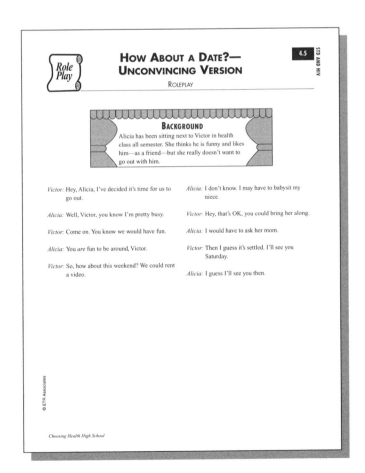

Role Play

HOW ABOUT A DATE?— UNCONVINCING VERSION

ROLEPLAY

4.5 | STD AND HIV

BACKGROUND

Alicia has been sitting next to Victor in health class all semester. She thinks he is funny and likes him—as a friend—but she really doesn't want to go out with him.

Victor: Hey, Alicia, I've decided it's time for us to go out.

Alicia: Well, Victor, you know I'm pretty busy.

Victor: Come on. You know we would have fun.

Alicia: You *are* fun to be around, Victor.

Victor: So, how about this weekend? We could rent a video.

Alicia: I don't know. I may have to babysit my niece.

Victor: Hey, that's OK, you could bring her along.

Alicia: I would have to ask her mom.

Victor: Then I guess it's settled. I'll see you Saturday.

Alicia: I guess I'll see you then.

© ETR Associates

Choosing Health High School

4. CONVINCING REFUSALS

CONTINUED

Roleplay effective refusals

Have the same 2 students read **How About a Date?—Convincing Version**. Again, read the Background section, then have the students present the roleplay. After the roleplay, ask the class to discuss what Alicia said and did that made her refusal convincing.

Ongoing Assessment Look for students' ability to identify the 5 parts of a convincing refusal:

- nonverbal no
- the word *no*
- repetition of the no message
- suggesting an alternate activity
- relationship building

SHARPEN THE SKILL
ASSERTIVENESS— HANDLING SITUATIONS

Explain that the refusals students are learning can be used in many different situations—for example, if a friend asks to borrow a favorite jacket or a sibling asks to borrow money. Have students suggest other examples. Allow them time to practice roleplaying assertiveness in these situations.

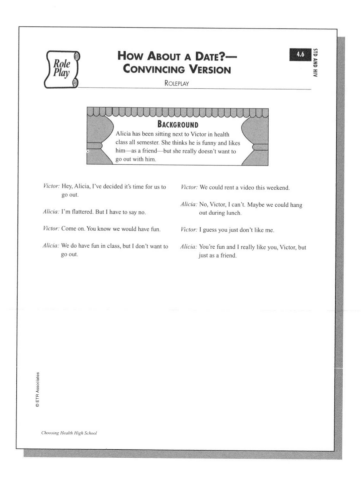

Role Play

HOW ABOUT A DATE?— CONVINCING VERSION

ROLEPLAY

4.6

STD AND HIV

BACKGROUND
Alicia has been sitting next to Victor in health class all semester. She thinks he is funny and likes him—as a friend—but she really doesn't want to go out with him.

Victor: Hey, Alicia, I've decided it's time for us to go out.

Alicia: I'm flattered. But I have to say no.

Victor: Come on. You know we would have fun.

Alicia: We do have fun in class, but I don't want to go out.

Victor: We could rent a video this weekend.

Alicia: No, Victor, I can't. Maybe we could hang out during lunch.

Victor: I guess you just don't like me.

Alicia: You're fun and I really like you, Victor, but just as a friend.

© ETR Associates

Choosing Health High School

EVALUATION

OBJECTIVE 1

Students will be able to:

> **Plan responses that reinforce the decision to be abstinent.**

Observe students' participation in the group discussion from Activity 2 and assess their responses on the **Handling** *Caution* **Situations** activity sheet for their ability to respond to *caution* situations in a way that promotes abstinence.

CRITERIA

See the **Following Through on Abstinence** *Instant Expert* for evaluation criteria.

(continued...)

REVIEW
- Following Through on Abstinence *Instant Expert* (p. 51)

MATERIALS
- completed Handling *Caution* Situations (4.2), from Activity 2

EVALUATION

10 minutes

✳

REVIEW

◆ Following Through on Abstinence
Instant Expert (p. 51)

MATERIALS

◆ Just This Once (4.7)

✳

OBJECTIVE 2

Students will be able to:

> **Recognize nonverbal and verbal refusal skills.**

    Distribute the **Just This Once** evaluation sheet. Have students complete the dialogue on the script using the skills for a convincing refusal.

CRITERIA

See the **Following Through on Abstinence** *Instant Expert* for evaluation criteria for convincing refusals.

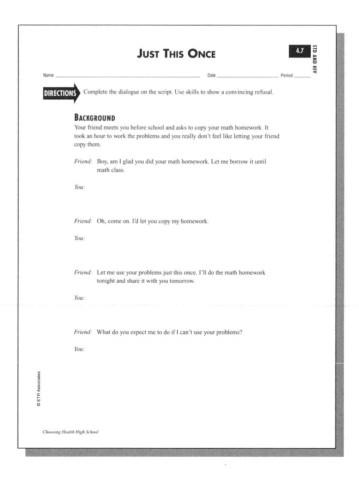

FOLLOWING THROUGH ON ABSTINENCE

Once a person has decided to be abstinent, follow-through is necessary. This involves thinking and planning to be successful. The following steps can help support a decision to be abstinent.

STEPS FOR FOLLOW-THROUGH

1. Talk with partners who might exert pressure to have intercourse. Explain personal feelings and beliefs. The best time to talk is not in the "heat of passion." Choose a calmer, more thoughtful time to talk, and plan what to say ahead of time.
2. Discuss ways, besides intercourse, to show feelings. Many different behaviors that show caring may be acceptable to both partners. Holding hands, kissing, putting arms around each other all express closeness and affection.
3. Find a variety of ways to be with a partner. Spending time with other friends and couples or activities such as tennis or other sports help keep a relationship "under control."
4. Make time for self and for friends other than a steady partner. Developing one's personality and abilities helps a person be well-rounded, and this benefits all of a person's relationships.
5. Be sensitive to situations that make it hard to stick to a decision to be abstinent.

DANGER AND *CAUTION* SITUATIONS

Situations that should be planned for or avoided fall into 2 categories:

Danger **situations** mean that a person is in a circumstance that may lead to sexual intercourse unless immediate action is taken. *Danger* situations usually occur when (1) a couple is alone and (2) they have done a lot of kissing and touching.

Examples of *danger* situations include:
- Touching each other in more ways.
- Getting sexually excited.
- Removing clothing.
- Lying down together.

Caution **situations** signal that a *danger* situation may be approaching. *Caution* situations occur when someone is planning or thinking about being with a girlfriend or boyfriend. When experiencing a *caution* situation, it is wise to plan ways to stick to the decision to be abstinent and to avoid a *danger* situation.

(continued...)

FOLLOWING THROUGH ON ABSTINENCE

Examples of *caution* situations include:
- Planning ways to be alone with a partner.
- Thinking about touching a partner.
- Planning to get and use alcohol or other drugs to relax.
- Dressing in a sexy way.

HANDLING SITUATIONS

The best way to handle a *caution* situation is to plan ways to avoid a *danger* situation. For example, people may notice that they are picking out sexy clothes to wear on a date. When they recognize this situation as a *caution* they can think about ways to avoid a *danger* situation. For example, they may decide to wear something different or think about things they can do on the date that will be fun but won't put them in a situation where they are alone with their boyfriend or girlfriend.

Most *danger* situations can be avoided if a person is alert to the *caution* situations that precede them. When *danger* situations do occur, *refusals* are required.

REFUSAL SKILLS

Refusals are a way to say no when a person does not want to have sex but values the relationship. Both verbal and nonverbal skills are involved in making a clear refusal.

What we say with our bodies and tone of voice is just as important as what we say with words. Here are some ways for people to communicate that they mean what they are saying:

- **erect posture**—Stand or sit erect and hold the head up to send a message of authority.
- **firm expression**—Look a partner in the eye, with an "I mean it" facial expression.
- **serious voice**—Use a strong and sincere tone.

There are 5 parts to a convincing refusal. The refusal should include:
- **a nonverbal no** (erect posture, firm expression, serious tone of voice)
- **the word** *no*
- **repetition of the no message** (as often as needed)
- **suggesting an alternate activity** (something else to do)
- **relationship building** (letting the other person know the relationship is valued)

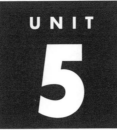

U N I T

5

USING REFUSALS

TIME
2 periods

ACTIVITIES
1. Remembering Refusals
2. Practicing Refusals
3. Practice Makes Perfect
4. Ad-Libbing Refusals

USING REFUSALS

OBJECTIVE

Students will be able to:

> Demonstrate refusals in roleplay situations.

GETTING STARTED

Have:

- transparency of **Refusals (4.4)**, from Unit 4

Copy for each student:

- Remembering Refusals (5.1)
- Skills for Refusals (5.2)
- Home Alone *Roleplay* (5.4)
- A Walk in the Park *Roleplay* (5.5)

Copy:

- Cookies and Yogurt *Roleplay* (5.3), 2 copies

UNIT OVERVIEW

PURPOSE

After refusals are modeled, students can begin practicing them. As with all skills, practice increases the likelihood that refusals will be used—in this case, to follow through on decisions to be abstinent.

MAIN POINTS

✳ Refusals can be used to say **no** to sex while maintaining a relationship.

✳ Practice enables a person to become more comfortable using refusals.

REVIEW

To increase your understanding about the importance of using and practicing refusals, review **Refusals in Relationships** *Instant Expert* (p. 61) and **Remembering Refusals Key** (p. 62).

1. REMEMBERING REFUSALS

A SELF-ASSESSMENT ACTIVITY

15 minutes

MATERIALS

◆ transparency of Refusals (4.4), from Unit 4
◆ Remembering Refusals (5.1)

Review refusals

Review the skills for refusals by displaying the **Refusals** transparency from Unit 4. Distribute a **Remembering Refusals** activity sheet to each student. Allow 5 minutes for students to complete the activity sheet.

Discuss responses

Have students correct their own sheets as the answers are discussed in class, using the **Remembering Refusals** *Key*. For Part 1, ask volunteers to identify which statements use skills for refusals and why. For Part 2, have volunteers share their statements and describe which of the skills they used.

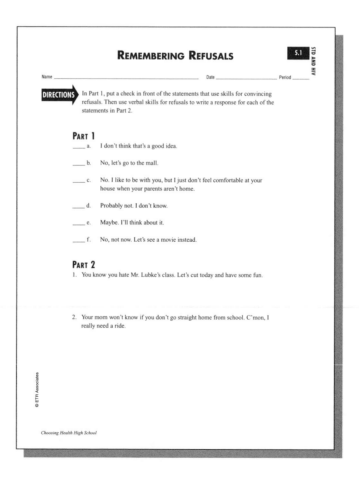

REMEMBERING REFUSALS 5.1 | STD AND HIV

Name _____ Date _____ Period _____

DIRECTIONS In Part 1, put a check in front of the statements that use skills for convincing refusals. Then use verbal skills for refusals to write a response for each of the statements in Part 2.

PART 1

____ a.   I don't think that's a good idea.

____ b.   No, let's go to the mall.

____ c.   No. I like to be with you, but I just don't feel comfortable at your house when your parents aren't home.

____ d.   Probably not. I don't know.

____ e.   Maybe. I'll think about it.

____ f.   No, not now. Let's see a movie instead.

PART 2

1.   You know you hate Mr. Lubke's class. Let's cut today and have some fun.

2.   Your mom won't know if you don't go straight home from school. C'mon, I really need a ride.

© ETR Associates

Choosing Health High School

2. PRACTICING REFUSALS

Demonstrate refusals

Distribute a **Skills for Refusals** activity sheet to each student and explain that it will be used as a checklist for the roleplays. Ask 2 student volunteers to act out the parts of the **Cookies and Yogurt** *Roleplay*. Instruct the class to put a check mark by each skill they observe being used in the roleplay. Read the Background section to set up the roleplay, then have the volunteers perform the script.

Identify skills

After the roleplay, review the skills that were used. Ask students to identify examples of the skills listed on the **Skills for Refusals** activity sheet.

Save the activity sheets for use in Activities 3 and 4.

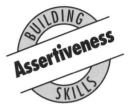

20 minutes

MATERIALS

- transparency of Refusals (4.4), from Unit 4
- Skills for Refusals (5.2)
- Cookies and Yogurt *Roleplay* (5.3)

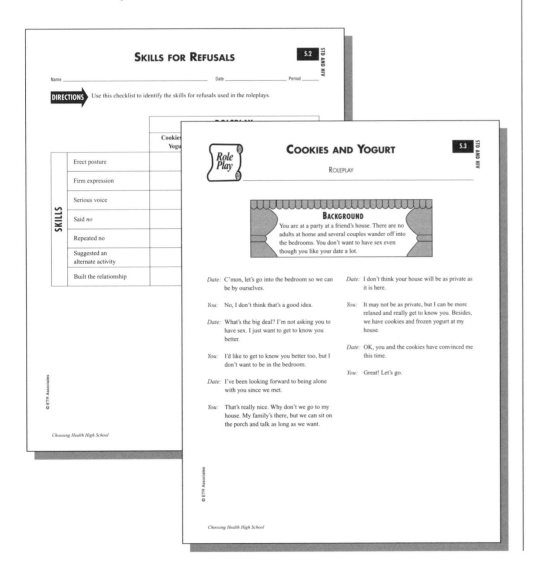

SKILLS FOR REFUSALS | 5.2 | STD AND HIV

Name _____ Date _____ Period _____

DIRECTIONS Use this checklist to identify the skills for refusals used in the roleplays.

SKILLS	
Erect posture	
Firm expression	
Serious voice	
Said *no*	
Repeated no	
Suggested an alternate activity	
Built the relationship	

© ETR Associates

Choosing Health High School

Role Play | **COOKIES AND YOGURT** | 5.3 | STD AND HIV

ROLEPLAY

BACKGROUND
You are at a party at a friend's house. There are no adults at home and several couples wander off into the bedrooms. You don't want to have sex even though you like your date a lot.

Date: C'mon, let's go into the bedroom so we can be by ourselves.

You: No, I don't think that's a good idea.

Date: What's the big deal? I'm not asking you to have sex. I just want to get to know you better.

You: I'd like to get to know you better too, but I don't want to be in the bedroom.

Date: I've been looking forward to being alone with you since we met.

You: That's really nice. Why don't we go to my house. My family's there, but we can sit on the porch and talk as long as we want.

Date: I don't think your house will be as private as it is here.

You: It may not be as private, but I can be more relaxed and really get to know you. Besides, we have cookies and frozen yogurt at my house.

Date: OK, you and the cookies have convinced me this time.

You: Great! Let's go.

© ETR Associates

Choosing Health High School

3. PRACTICE MAKES PERFECT

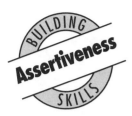

BUILDING *Assertiveness* **SKILLS**

25 minutes

✹

MATERIALS

♦ Skills for Refusals (5.2), from Activity 2

♦ Home Alone *Roleplay* (5.4)

✹

MEETING STUDENT NEEDS

It may be necessary to designate who in each triad will be first to read a script, who will serve as the first observer, etc. Circulate around the room and guide the rotation process.

✹

Triads practice refusals

Distribute the **Home Alone** *Roleplay*. Give students 5 minutes to finish the script. Divide students into groups of 3. Explain that they will act out their scripts and observe the roleplays.

Instruct students to rotate within their groups, reading their own script (author), reading a partner's script (reader) and serving as the observer. (In the next rotation, the author becomes the observer, the reader becomes the author and the observer becomes the reader.)

The observer is to use his or her **Skills for Refusals** activity sheet to check the skills used in the roleplay. After each rotation, the groups will use the observer's activity sheet to discuss the skills that were used.

Discuss the roleplays

When the 3 rotations are finished, have students discuss the experience as a class. Points for discussion include:

• ease or difficulty in using the skills
• skills that are easiest to use
• situations where refusals could be used

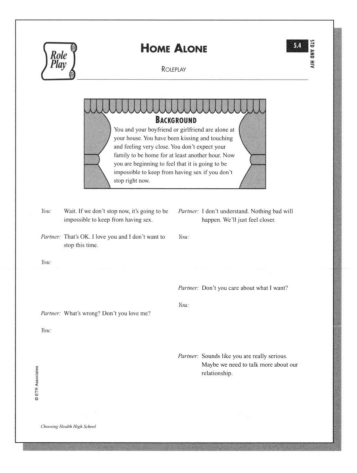

4. AD-LIBBING REFUSALS

Triads ad-lib refusals

Pass out the **A Walk in the Park** *Roleplay*, which presents an unscripted scenario. Divide students into groups of 3. Explain that this time they will practice refusals by ad-libbing responses instead of writing out their scripts. They should act as if this is a real scene and they have to rely on what they have learned about refusals.

Have students rotate within their groups so that each person has an opportunity to read the part of the date, ad-lib the responses and serve as the observer. The observer should use his or her **Skills for Refusals** activity sheet to check the skills as they are used in the roleplay. After each rotation, the groups will use the observer's activity sheet to discuss the skills that were used.

Discuss and share roleplays

When groups are finished, reassemble the class to discuss the experience. Ask volunteers to roleplay some of the scripts they ad-libbed in their triads. Have the class use the **Skills for Refusals** activity sheet to identify and discuss the skills used.

20 minutes

MATERIALS

- Skills for Refusals (5.2), from Activity 2
- A Walk in the Park *Roleplay* (5.5)

EXTEND THE LEARNING

Have students discuss whether the roleplays (**Cookies and Yogurt**, **Home Alone** and **A Walk in the Park**) are examples of *caution* or *danger* situations.

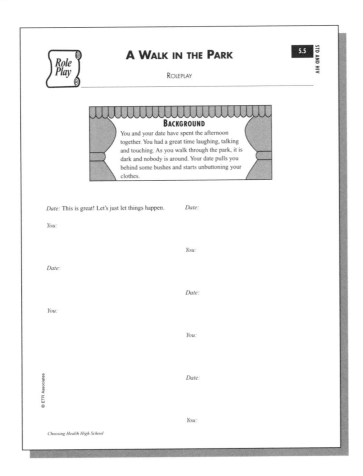

Role Play

A WALK IN THE PARK

5.5 STD AND HIV

ROLEPLAY

BACKGROUND

You and your date have spent the afternoon together. You had a great time laughing, talking and touching. As you walk through the park, it is dark and nobody is around. Your date pulls you behind some bushes and starts unbuttoning your clothes.

Date: This is great! Let's just let things happen.

You:

Date:

You:

Date:

Date:

You:

You:

Date:

You:

© ETR Associates

Choosing Health High School

EVALUATION

OBJECTIVE

Students will be able to:

Demonstrate refusals in roleplay situations.

Observe students' participation in group roleplays during Activities 3 and 4 for their ability to use nonverbal and verbal refusal skills.

CRITERIA

Assess the roleplay practice in groups and class discussion for students' ability to demonstrate:

- erect posture
- firm expression
- serious voice
- use of the word *no*
- repetition of the no message
- an alternate suggestion
- relationship building

REFUSALS IN RELATIONSHIPS

Refusals are difficult within relationships people value. It is much more difficult for people to say no when they care about another person and want to continue being close than to say no to a stranger or an acquaintance. Also, many cultures teach children and young adults to be as accommodating and helpful as possible. This cultural training may make refusals even more difficult.

In some encounters, saying no to sex is all that is required. But when a partner desires intercourse and the relationship is at stake, suggesting alternate activities and relationship building are invaluable. An individual may not need to include every skill in each refusal; but it is a good idea to practice as many of the skills as possible to get accustomed to using them.

Young people need to feel empowered to say no when they have made the decision to be abstinent. As with all skills, practice allows students to feel more comfortable saying no and increases the probability that this skill will be used in *caution* or *danger* situations. The more students practice and use refusals, the more refusal skills become part of their repertoire.

REMEMBERING REFUSALS

KEY

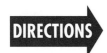 **DIRECTIONS** In Part 1, put a check in front of the statements that use skills for convincing refusals. Then use verbal skills for refusals to write a response for each of the statements in Part 2.

PART 1

____ a.   I don't think that's a good idea.

✔ b.   No, let's go to the mall. *(used the word no, suggested an alternate activity)*

✔ c.   No. I like to be with you, but I just don't feel comfortable at your house when your parents aren't home. *(used the word no, built the relationship)*

____ d.   Probably not. I don't know.

____ e.   Maybe. I'll think about it.

✔ f.   No, not now. Let's see a movie instead. *(used the word no, suggested an alternate activity)*

PART 2

1.   You know you hate Mr. Lubke's class. Let's cut today and have some fun.
   No, I don't hate Mr. Lubke's class enough to get detention. Let's plan to do something fun after school tomorrow.

2.   Your mom won't know if you don't go straight home from school. C'mon, I really need a ride.
   No, I've got to get home but let's ask Tamra if she can give you a ride. She lives in your neighborhood.

PROTECTION WITH A CAPITAL C

TIME

2 periods

ACTIVITIES

1. Risky Behaviors

2. Let's Talk

3. Condom Communication

4. Information About Condoms

5. The Cost of Condoms

6. Encouraging Condom Use

PROTECTION WITH A CAPITAL C

OBJECTIVES

Students will be able to:

1. Demonstrate ways to talk to a partner about using condoms.

2. Explain steps for male condom use.

3. Survey products that provide protection from STD.

GETTING STARTED

Have:

- tagboard
- envelopes
- unlined paper
- colored pencils or markers
- glue
- clip art or magazines

Copy 1 for each group:
- Let's Talk (6.1)
- Steps for Condom Use (6.3)

Copy for each student:
- Condom Communication (6.2)
- Pricing Protection Products (6.4)

SPECIAL STEPS

Prepare **Steps for Condom Use** tagboard strips and envelopes for student groups. See Activity 4 (p. 70).

UNIT OVERVIEW

PURPOSE

In order to use condoms effectively, teens must understand the steps for correct usage. Additionally, they must be motivated to use protection. By addressing factors related to condom use, sexually active teens will be more likely to protect themselves from STD.

MAIN POINTS

✳ Partners can and should discuss using protection before having sexual intercourse.

✳ Condoms must be used correctly in order to provide protection from STD.

✳ Products that provide protection from STD are accessible to teens.

REVIEW

To increase your understanding of condom use, review *Teaching About Condom Use Instant Expert* (p. 75).

VOCABULARY

ejaculation—The expulsion of semen from the penis.

female condom—A polyurethane pouch inserted into the vagina to prevent the exchange of body fluids.

male condom—A covering stretched over the penis to prevent the exchange of body fluids.

nonoxynol-9—A chemical that kills sperm and may help protect against the pathogens that cause some STD.

1. RISKY BEHAVIORS

10 minutes

✳

EXTEND THE LEARNING

Discuss the issues of risk in a broader sense. Have students look up the meaning of *risk*. Ask them to identify examples of risky behaviors teens may be engaged in that are not related to sex.

✳

Brainstorm reasons for risky behaviors

Conduct a brainstorming session to identify reasons teens engage in risky sexual behaviors even though they know about "no-risk" and "protection" behaviors. Examples:

- embarrassed to discuss with partner
- embarrassed to buy condoms and spermicides
- partner doesn't want to practice "no-risk" or "protection" behaviors
- don't think they are at risk
- don't have money to buy condoms
- don't like the way condoms feel
- under the influence of alcohol and/or other drugs

Brainstorm ways to be comfortable with condoms

Conduct a brainstorming session to identify what teens could do to become more comfortable with using condoms. Examples:

- practice putting on and taking off condoms while alone
- learn more about condoms
- talk to their partner

2. LET'S TALK

Groups brainstorm topics

Divide students into small groups. Distribute a Let's Talk activity sheet to each group. Ask groups to brainstorm topics a couple should talk about before they have sex and add the most important ones to the activity sheet. Instruct the groups to put all the topics in order by writing a "1" beside the topic that is easiest to talk about, a "2" by the topic that is next, etc. They should try to achieve consensus on the ranking within the group.

Discuss communication about using condoms

Ask groups to share the topics they added to their lists and the order in which they put the topics. Discuss the ranking of topics that involve the use of condoms. Focus the discussion on the importance of talking about condoms and why talking about condoms may be difficult.

15 minutes

MATERIALS

♦ Let's Talk (6.1)

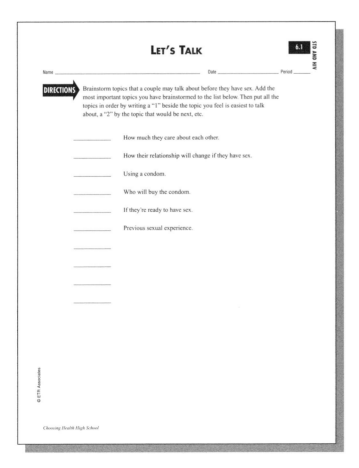

LET'S TALK   6.1   STD AND HIV

Name _____ Date _____ Period _____

DIRECTIONS Brainstorm topics that a couple may talk about before they have sex. Add the most important topics you have brainstormed to the list below. Then put all the topics in order by writing a "1" beside the topic you feel is easiest to talk about, a "2" by the topic that would be next, etc.

_____ How much they care about each other.

_____ How their relationship will change if they have sex.

_____ Using a condom.

_____ Who will buy the condom.

_____ If they're ready to have sex.

_____ Previous sexual experience.

_____

_____

_____

_____

© ETR Associates

Choosing Health High School

3. CONDOM COMMUNICATION

A ROLEPLAY ACTIVITY

20 minutes

✴

MATERIALS

◆ Condom Communication (6.2)

✴

EXTEND THE LEARNING

Set up a debate in which students take a stand about availability of condoms. Have them present their arguments verbally or in writing. For example, post the following question: Should companies that make condoms be allowed to advertise their product on TV? Why or why not?

✴

Class brainstorms ways to talk about condoms

Have the class brainstorm things teens could say to introduce condom use into a conversation. Examples:

- "There's something I've been wanting us to talk about—I think we should use a condom."
- "You know how much I care about you. I want to protect you by using a condom."

Emphasize that the dialogue should be direct yet sensitive to the feelings of both partners.

Write the ideas on the board and ask students to consider what dialogue would feel most comfortable to them. Also ask students to consider how they would feel if a partner said these statements to them.

(continued…)

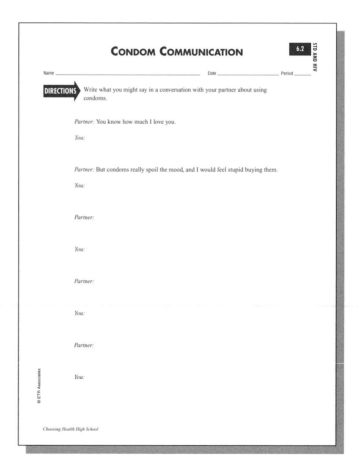

3. CONDOM COMMUNICATION

(CONTINUED)

Students complete roleplay scripts

Distribute a **Condom Communication** activity sheet to each student. Ask students to complete the script. They can begin the dialogue by using some of the statements that were brainstormed or they can create all new dialogue. Instruct students to discuss condom use in a direct and sensitive way. They should address the importance of using a condom and who will buy the condoms.

After students have completed their scripts, ask for volunteers to choose a partner and read their scripts. Ask the rest of the class to provide feedback after the scripts are read.

Ongoing Assessment Student feedback about the roleplay scripts should focus on:

- Direct dialogue (Are condoms and reasons to use them discussed? Who will buy them?)
- Sensitivity to the partner's feelings (addressing his or her concerns)

COMMUNITY LINK

Ask students to recall a movie, video or television program that portrayed a couple who has a sexual relationship. Focus discussion on whether or not the couple discussed STD or using protection. Have students consider the ways in which media portray sexual relationships. Are these realistic?

4. Information About Condoms

25 minutes

MATERIALS

♦ prepared Steps for Condom Use tagboard strips and envelopes

---

Discuss how to use condoms

Discuss condom use, using the **Teaching About Condom Use** *Instant Expert* as a guide. Explain the 7 steps for using male condoms. Allow time for questions and discussion.

Groups unscramble steps

Scramble and display the tagboard strips with the **Steps for Condom Use**. Ask students to choose 2 partners to work with to unscramble the 7 steps. Give each triad an envelope containing the prepared **Steps for Condom Use**. Ask groups to unscramble the steps and put them in the correct order.

Rearrange tagboard strips

Ask 1 triad to volunteer to arrange the tagboard strips in the correct order. Point out the emphasized letter in each of the 7 steps. Note that the letters spell *protect*.

(continued...)

STEPS FOR CONDOM USE

Print the **Steps for Condom Use** on separate strips of tagboard. Print the capitalized letters that spell "protect" in a different color for added emphasis.

Make a copy of the **Steps for Condom Use (6.3)** for each group of 3 students. Cut the strips apart and place each set of strips in an envelope.

Discuss using condoms with **P**artner.
Open the package and **R**emove the condom carefully.
Unr**O**ll the condom onto the erect penis, leaving 1/2 inch at the tip.
Add lubrica**T**ion.
Hold the rim of the condom in place when withdrawing the p**E**nis.
Take off the **C**ondom away from partner's genitals.
Throw the used condom away.

---

4. INFORMATION ABOUT CONDOMS

(CONTINUED)

Discuss condom use

Remind students that condom use is a "protection" behavior, and that it requires thought and planning. Ask students:

- What are some situations that might lead to poor decisions about condom use? (When you are in the middle of heavy petting or under the influence of alcohol.)
- When is a good time to make a decision about condom use? (While you are not under pressure and can think carefully. When you can discuss it with your partner.)

Discuss the kinds of things that would encourage teens to use condoms. Examples:

- believing they are at risk
- having a partner who wants to practice "preventive" behaviors
- believing behavior can protect from STD
- knowing someone who has an STD
- caring about a partner
- knowing how to use condoms

Students write reasons for condom use

Ask students to work with triad partners to identify 2 reasons why sexually active teens should use condoms. Have them write down the reasons.

Discuss reasons

Have triads report their reasons for condom use. Summarize the reasons students have listed.

(Ongoing Assessment) Look for students' ability to identify reasons to use condoms. Reasons might include:

- protection from STD
- protection from unintended pregnancy
- responsible behavior for self and others

MEETING STUDENT NEEDS

Students can benefit from seeing a demonstration of condom use if state and local guidelines permit. Condom use can be demonstrated using a penis model, zucchini or banana, or the index and middle fingers of your hand. You may want to ask the school nurse or a community health educator to provide this demonstration.

5. THE COST OF CONDOMS

10 minutes

MATERIALS

♦ Pricing Protection Products (6.4)

MEETING STUDENT NEEDS

Make sure this activity fits within district guidelines. Be sensitive to the fact that this is a challenging and potentially embarrassing activity for some students. Modify the activity to meet the needs of your class.

Students survey prices

Distribute the **Pricing Protection Products** activity sheet. Ask students to visit a store where condoms and/or products containing nonoxynol-9 are sold and to answer the questions on the activity sheet.

Students report

Have students report their findings to the class. Discuss the information.

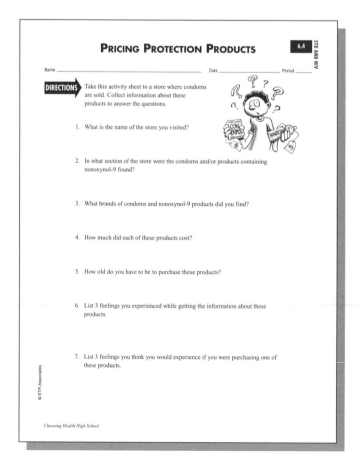

6. ENCOURAGING CONDOM USE

Groups develop pamphlets

Have students work in small groups to develop a pamphlet. Make art supplies available to groups and explain the pamphlet requirements:

- Describe the steps for condom use. Illustrate them if you choose.
- Provide information about discussing condom use with a partner.
- Describe how to access condoms and products containing nonoxynol-9 (where to buy, price, etc.).
- Include any other information you feel is important.
- Give your pamphlet a title.

Ongoing Assessment Pamphlets should include the correct steps for condom use, ideas for discussing condoms with a partner, and how to access protection. You may also assess student work for attractiveness, readability, use of art and spelling and grammar.

25 minutes

MATERIALS

- unlined paper
- colored pencils or markers
- glue
- clip art or magazines

EXTEND THE LEARNING

Students could use a computer with a program that contains graphics to produce and print the pamphlet.

EVALUATION

MATERIALS

♦ completed Condom Communication (6.2), from Activity 3

REVIEW

♦ Teaching About Condom Use *Instant Expert* (p. 75)

MATERIALS

♦ completed student pamphlets, from Activity 6

MATERIALS

♦ completed Pricing Protection Products (6.4), from Activity 5

OBJECTIVE 1

Students will be able to:

> **Demonstrate ways to talk to a partner about using condoms.**

Assess students' **Condom Communication** activity sheets for their ability to create dialogue that discusses condom use.

CRITERIA

Activity sheets should contain dialogue that is direct and sensitive to the feelings of both partners.

OBJECTIVE 2

Students will be able to:

> **Explain steps for male condom use.**

Assess groups' work in sorting the Steps for Condom Use in Activity 4 and students' pamphlets from Activity 6 for their ability to explain the steps.

CRITERIA

Look for correct order of the 7 steps for male condom use. See **Teaching About Condom Use** *Instant Expert* for evaluation criteria.

OBJECTIVE 3

Students will be able to:

> **Survey products that provide protection from STD.**

Observe students' participation in class reports and assess their responses on the **Pricing Protection Products** activity sheet for their ability to gather information about products that provide protection from STD.

CRITERIA

Students should be able to describe:

• Products that provide protection.
• Where protection products can be purchased.
• The cost of condoms and products containing nonoxynol-9.

TEACHING ABOUT CONDOM USE

Abstinence and mutual monogamy with an uninfected partner are "no-risk" behaviors, but not all teenagers will choose them. For teens who are sexually active, latex condoms used with products containing nonoxynol-9 are the best protection against STD. Over 50% of high school students report being sexually active; these teens need information about correct condom use.

GUIDELINES FOR TEACHING CONDOM USE

Educators must become acquainted with guidelines established in their school or community for teaching this material and select their teaching approaches accordingly. Be as explicit as possible given the setting. Be prepared to accept some laughter and embarrassment during the condom lesson. Consider taking time to address the reactions and feelings students have about condoms.

Various approaches can be used to teach condom use, such as verbal or visual instruction or a demonstration.

Verbal Instruction

When using verbal instruction, some educators prefer the passive voice for discussing condom use. For example, "Condoms are more effective when used with birth control foam" (passive voice), rather than "Use birth control foam when you use a condom" (active voice). Passive voice is less likely to be interpreted as an endorsement for teen sexual activity. When using verbal instruction, be sure students understand the basic anatomy and physiology necessary for condom use.

Visual Instruction

Visual instruction can be combined with verbal instruction. Brochures, pictures or transparencies are used to illustrate the steps of condom use. If possible, it is helpful to display condoms for students to examine or to have one to show them.

Demonstration

Demonstration of condoms is different from displaying and examining condoms. Demonstration of male condom use should be practiced beforehand. One simple method for demonstration consists of unwrapping a condom and unrolling it over the index and middle finger of the hand. Some educators use cucumbers, bananas or models of the penis to illustrate condom use. *It is particularly important to familiarize yourself with district guidelines for demonstrations of condom use, because they differ greatly among school districts.*

(continued...)

TEACHING ABOUT CONDOM USE

CORRECT CONDOM USE

Condoms work by providing a barrier that prevents the direct contact of mucous membranes and the exchange of body fluids. While condoms are easy to use, they are not foolproof. They must be used properly to be effective. Proper use means a new condom has to be used every time a couple has sexual intercourse, from start to finish. Even when condoms are used correctly, they are not 100% effective.

It is important to practice using a condom before and without having intercourse. Practice allows the user to get familiar with how to place the condom correctly, and how the condom looks and feels.

Condoms should be stored in a cool, dry place and discarded if not used before the expiration date. They should not be kept in a wallet or car where heat and sunlight can weaken them. Women as well as men should carry condoms.

Products that contain nonoxynol-9 (contraceptive foams, creams, suppositories, films and jellies) have been shown to kill some of the pathogens that cause STD. Using one of these products with a condom provides additional protection, although some people may be allergic to nonoxynol-9. Oil-based lubricants, such as petroleum jelly, baby oil or cold cream should *never* be used with condoms. These lubricants weaken the condom and may cause it to break.

Male Condom

For males, latex rather than "natural membrane" condoms should be used. The word *latex* will appear on the package. Natural membrane condoms have larger pores and may not be as effective in blocking pathogens. Most grocery stores, drug stores and health clinics sell condoms of good quality.

The condom should always be put on as soon as the penis is erect and hard. Small drops of pre-ejaculate fluid come out of the penis before orgasm, and this fluid can contain pathogens as well as sperm.

Latex condoms for males are very effective at preventing STD if used properly.

Female Condom

If a male condom is not going to be used during intercourse, a woman can protect herself by using a female condom. The female condom cannot be used with a male condom because the condoms will not stay in place when used together.

The female condom is a soft, loose-fitting plastic pouch that lines the vagina. It has a ring at each end. One ring is used to put the condom inside the vagina and hold it in place. The other ring stays outside the vagina and partly covers the vulva.

(continued…)

TEACHING ABOUT CONDOM USE

A female condom can be inserted up to 8 hours before sexual intercourse; however, most women insert the condom several minutes before having sex.

STEPS FOR CORRECT MALE CONDOM USE

To use a condom properly, these 7 steps should be followed:

1. Discuss using condoms. This discussion should occur between the partners in a relaxed and open atmosphere.

2. Open the package carefully and remove the condom. Handle the condom gently to avoid tearing it. Be particularly careful of fingernails and jewelry that could damage the latex.

3. Unroll the condom onto the erect penis, all the way down to the base. Pinch the tip of the condom to keep air out and leave about 1/2 inch of room at the tip. If there is no room for semen at the tip, the condom may break.

4. Add lubrication. Products that contain nonoxynol-9 are the best. Avoid products that contain oil (petroleum jelly, baby oil, cold cream). These products weaken the latex and can cause it to break. Some condoms are prelubricated.

5. Hold the rim of the condom in place when withdrawing the penis. Remove the penis from partner's body immediately after ejaculation, before the penis begins to become flaccid. Holding onto the rim keeps the condom from slipping off while withdrawing.

6. Take off the condom away from partner's genitals.

7. Throw the used condom away. Never reuse a condom.

STD SYMPTOMS, CONSEQUENCES AND TREATMENT

TIME

2–3 periods

ACTIVITIES

1. STD Symptoms

2. Symptoms and Consequences

3. Being Informed

4. Diagnosis and Treatment

5. STD Sleuth

STD Symptoms, Consequences and Treatment

OBJECTIVES

Students will be able to:

> 1. Describe symptoms and consequences of STD.

> 2. Identify and utilize sources for obtaining information, diagnosis and treatment of STD.

GETTING STARTED

Have:

- 6 envelopes

Copy a classroom set of:
- STD Symptoms and Consequences (7.1)

Copy 1 for each group:
- Rosa and Ramon *Case Study* (7.2)   • Frederick *Case Study* (7.4)
- Melissa and Josh *Case Study* (7.3)   • Michael and Sunny *Case Study* (7.5)

Copy for each student:
- Finding Information About STD (7.6)

Copy:
- STD Sleuth Clues (7.7)

SPECIAL STEPS

Prepare an STD Hotlines and Clinics classroom display. See Activity 3 (p. 85).

Prepare clue envelopes for STD Sleuth Game. See Activity 5 (p. 88).

UNIT OVERVIEW

PURPOSE

With an understanding of STD symptoms and consequences, students are more motivated to seek treatment. This lesson focuses on symptoms that may indicate the presence of STD, health consequences that may arise as the result of infection, and resources that supply STD diagnosis and treatment.

MAIN POINTS

* Symptoms can alert people to the possibility that they may have an STD.
* A person can have an STD and have *no* symptoms.
* Some STDs can be cured.
* HIV, herpes and genital warts are 3 STDs that cannot be cured.
* Early treatment of most STD can prevent serious health consequences.
* Many agencies and organizations provide information, diagnosis and treatment related to STD.

REVIEW

To increase your understanding of symptoms and treatment of STD, review **STD Symptoms and Treatment** *Instant Expert* (p. 90) and the **STD Case Studies Key** (p. 93).

VOCABULARY

abstinence—Avoiding sexual intercourse.

chlamydia—Common STD, caused by bacteria.

effect—Something brought about by a cause.

genital warts—An STD that causes small, bumpy warts on the sex organs or anus.

gonorrhea—Common STD, caused by bacteria.

herpes simplex—A virus associated with sores either around the mouth and lips or on the genitals.

HIV—Human immunodeficiency virus; the virus that causes AIDS.

infectious agent—A microorganism that causes disease.

intercourse—A type of sexual contact.

NGU—Nongonococcal urethritis; an STD with symptoms similar to gonorrhea.

perinatal transmission—Passing an infection to a baby during birth.

prenatal transmission—Passing an infection to a fetus before birth.

prevention—Hindering something from happening or existing.

pubic lice—Parasites that live in pubic hair, armpits or eyebrows and cause itching.

sexually transmitted disease (STD)—Any of a number of infectious diseases spread through sexual contact.

symptoms—Indications of the presence of disease.

syphilis—An STD, caused by bacteria.

transmission—The passing of infection from 1 person to another.

treatment—Care to reduce symptoms, cure a disease or change a condition.

1. STD SYMPTOMS

20 minutes

✷

MATERIALS

♦ classroom set of STD Symptoms and Consequences (7.1)

✷

Read case study

Read "The Blind Date" case study to the class. Ask students to listen for the events and symptoms that provide clues to Henry's health problem.

Discuss case study

Discuss what Henry's symptoms might mean. Ask students questions such as the following:

- What do you think is wrong with Henry? (He may have an STD.)
- If Henry has an STD, in what behavior must he have participated? (sexual intercourse)

Students identify symptoms

Distribute the STD Symptoms and Consequences student reading page. Have students locate Henry's symptoms in the reading and identify which STDs cause these symptoms (chlamydia or gonorrhea). Ask students to look at the *Consequences* column on the chart to see what may happen to Henry if he doesn't get treated.

Discuss symptoms and consequences, using the STD Symptoms and Treatment *Instant Expert* as a guide. Ask students:

- Should Henry tell his steady girlfriend about the STD?
- How can Henry get tested and treated?

Collect the student reading pages for reuse.

THE BLIND DATE

Case Study

Henry had looked forward to visiting his cousin, Warren, for several months. They had practically grown up together, but had not seen much of each other since Warren's family moved away 2 years before. As soon as Henry arrived, Warren excitedly told him there would be a party that night and that he had arranged a blind date for Henry.

Henry enjoyed the party and had a great time with his date. Two weeks later, after he was home, Henry noticed a white discharge from his penis and felt pain when he urinated.

1. STD Symptoms

CONTINUED

Ongoing Assessment Look for students to be able to identify chlamydia or gonorrhea as the STDs that might cause Henry's symptoms. Consequences of not being treated include:

- giving the STD to other sexual partner(s)
- damage to reproductive organs
- sterility
- development of heart trouble, blindness, skin disease or arthritis

Students should also understand that if Henry and his steady girlfriend have engaged in sexual intercourse, she should be told. Women often do *not* have symptoms when they are infected.

Sources of information Henry could use to get help include:

- an STD hotline
- a personal physician
- a local STD clinic

EXTEND THE LEARNING

Have students develop posters or other informational items about how to get accurate information or help in regard to STD.

STD SYMPTOMS AND CONSEQUENCES　7.1

STUDENT READING

STD	SYMPTOMS	CONSEQUENCES
HIV	Symptoms begin several months to several years after infection. • Flu-like feelings that persist • Unexplained weight loss • Night sweats • Persistent diarrhea • White spots in mouth • Unexplained fatigue	You can give HIV to your sexual partner or someone you share a needle with. HIV cannot be cured. Many people die from it. HIV damages the immune system, making a person susceptible to many different illnesses and infections. Passed from mother to child before, during or after birth (through breastfeeding).
CHLAMYDIA	Symptoms begin 7–21 days after infection. • Most women and some men have no symptoms • Discharge from the sex organs • Burning or pain while urinating • Unusual bleeding from the vagina • Pain in the pelvic area	You can give chlamydia to your sexual partner. Can damage reproductive organs. Can cause sterility. Passed from mother to child during childbirth.
GENITAL WARTS	Symptoms begin 1–6 months after infection. • Small, bumpy warts on and around the sex organs • Itching and burning around the sex organs	You can give genital warts to your sexual partner. More warts can grow. Warts may signal precancerous condition. Passed from mother to child during childbirth.

© ETR Associates

(continued...)

Choosing Health High School

2. SYMPTOMS AND CONSEQUENCES

25 minutes

MATERIALS

- classroom set of STD Symptoms and Consequences (7.1)
- Rosa and Ramon, Melissa and Josh, Frederick, and Michael and Sunny *Case Studies* (7.2)–(7.5)

Groups analyze case studies

Divide students into 4 groups. Give each group a copy of 1 of the *Case Studies* and an **STD Symptoms and Consequences** student reading page. Explain the group assignment:

- Read the case study.
- Use information on the **STD Symptoms and Consequences** student reading page to answer the questions that follow each case study.

Discuss case studies

Discuss group work on the case studies and correct any misconceptions, using the **STD Case Studies** *Key* as a guide.

Collect the student reading pages for reuse.

Ongoing Assessment See the **STD Case Studies** *Key* for assessment criteria. Allow groups to redo and resubmit their work if students have not yet achieved the objective.

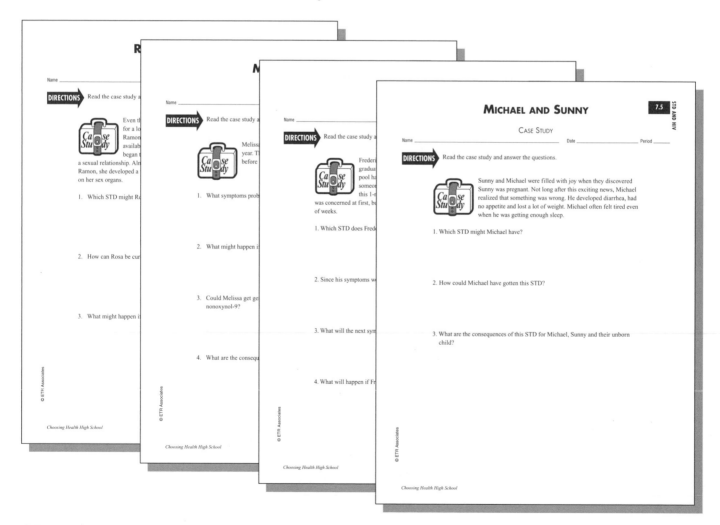

3. BEING INFORMED

Students research agencies

Divide students into groups of 4–5 and distribute the **Finding Information About STD** activity sheet. Point out the display of information about hotlines and local clinics and agencies. Ask students to fill in the hotline numbers on questions 2 and 5 and the name, address and phone number for a local clinic on question 9. Divide responsibilities for calling among the groups so hotlines and local clinics are not overwhelmed by student calls. Allow students time to complete the activity sheet out of class.

(continued...)

15 minutes

❊

MATERIALS

- Finding Information About STD (7.6)
- STD Hotlines and Clinics classroom display

❊

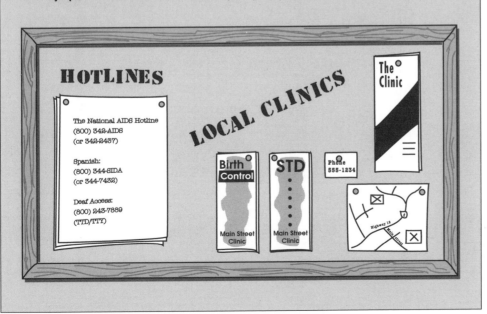

STD HOTLINES AND CLINICS CLASSROOM DISPLAY

Prepare a display with the names and phone numbers of local and national STD/HIV hotlines and information on local STD clinics or agencies. Use the Hotlines section of the **STD Symptoms and Treatment** *Instant Expert* (p. 90) as a resource.

3. BEING INFORMED

Discuss information sources

Ask groups who called hotlines to report on:

- the hotline name
- the questions they asked
- the answers to the questions
- how they felt calling the hotline
- the helpfulness and courtesy of the person answering the phone line

Have groups who called the local clinic report on:

- the name of the clinic
- the services offered
- the office hours
- the costs for STD testing and treatment
- whether services are confidential

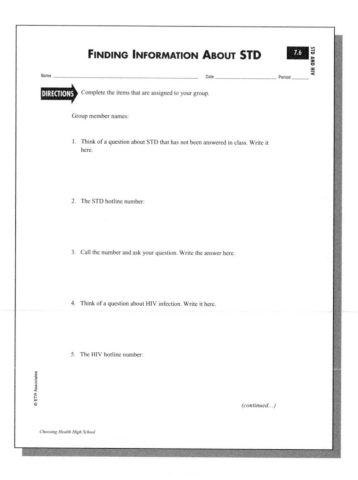

FINDING INFORMATION ABOUT STD　7.6　STD AND HIV

Name _____   Date _____   Period _____

DIRECTIONS　Complete the items that are assigned to your group.

Group member names:

1. Think of a question about STD that has not been answered in class. Write it here.

2. The STD hotline number:

3. Call the number and ask your question. Write the answer here.

4. Think of a question about HIV infection. Write it here.

5. The HIV hotline number:

© ETR Associates

(continued...)

Choosing Health High School

4. DIAGNOSIS AND TREATMENT

25 minutes

A CLASS DISCUSSION ACTIVITY

Discuss diagnosis and treatment

Discuss the diagnosis and treatment of STD, using the **STD Symptoms and Treatment** *Instant Expert* as a guide. Emphasize the following points:

- It's important to get tested and treated immediately.
- Treatments for STD are determined by the type of STD.

Ask students:

- What advice would you give someone who had a personal question about STD?
- What advice would you give someone who suspected he or she had become infected with an STD?

COMMUNITY LINK

Invite a health worker from a local clinic to speak to the class about the diagnosis and treatment of STD. Ask the speaker to include information about procedures for STD checkups, tests, physical exams, treatments and local incidence rates.

Or you could arrange to have a health worker stage a mock interview with a client who suspects she or he has an STD. Tape the interview to be played for the class.

5. STD Sleuth

20 minutes

MATERIALS

- prepared clue envelopes
- *Optional:* classroom set of STD Symptoms and Consequences (7.1)

Prepare for the game

Divide students into 5 teams. Explain that each team will receive an envelope containing clues to the identity of several types of STD. Their job is to trade clues with other teams until they have a set that describes a single STD. Distribute clue envelopes and explain the rules for the STD Sleuth Game.

Students play game

Signal teams to begin the game. Circulate around the room to monitor teams' progress.

Discuss game

Once all teams have finished, have each team read all their clues to the class and announce the name of the STD the clues describe.

STD SLEUTH GAME

Preparation

1. Copy the **STD Sleuth Clues** teacher page and cut apart the clue strips.
2. Distribute the strips among 5 envelopes. Each envelope should have 4 clues in it. Be sure that no envelope contains more than 2 clues for the same STD.

Rules for the Game

- Only 1 student at a time can leave the group to trade.
- No team is required to trade.
- Students may use any classroom resource to locate information. *(Note:* You might want to make the **STD Symptoms and Consequences** student reading page available.)
- The first team to collect all 4 clues for an STD is the winner.
- All teams must finish.

EVALUATION

OBJECTIVE 1

Students will be able to:

> **Describe symptoms and consequences of STD.**

Assess students' participation in class discussion in Activity 1 and their group work on the *Case Studies* activity sheets for their ability to describe consequences of STD infection.

CRITERIA

Look for accurate descriptions of consequences related to specific STDs. See the **STD Symptoms and Treatment** *Instant Expert,* the **STD Symptoms and Consequences** student reading page, and the **STD Case Studies** *Key* for evaluation criteria.

REVIEW

- STD Symptoms and Treatment *Instant Expert* (p. 90)
- STD Case Studies *Key* (p. 93)
- STD Symptoms and Consequences (7.1)

MATERIALS

- completed *Case Studies* (7.2–7.5), from Activity 2

OBJECTIVE 2

Students will be able to:

> **Identify and utilize sources for obtaining information, diagnosis and treatment of STD.**

Assess student responses on the **Finding Information About STD** activity sheet and in class discussion in Activity 4 for their ability to identify appropriate resources for STD information and treatment.

CRITERIA

Look for students to successfully contact STD hotlines or local resources for answers to their questions, and to suggest going to a clinic or health care provider if STD infection is suspected.

REVIEW

- STD Symptoms and Treatment *Instant Expert* (p. 90)

MATERIALS

- completed Finding Information About STD (7.6), from Activity 3

STD Symptoms and Treatment

Prompt treatment of STD is crucial. Untreated STD can lead to both short and long-term health consequences. An individual who is sexually active and who experiences 1 or more of the signs and symptoms of STD should be tested for STD. Through specific tests, medical providers can identify the disease and prescribe appropriate treatment.

SIGNS AND SYMPTOMS

Signs and symptoms that may indicate an STD include:

- an unusual discharge or odor from the sex organs
- sores, blisters or bumps near the sex organs or mouth
- pain or burning during urination or bowel movements
- pain in the pelvic area (lower abdomen)
- pain during sexual intercourse
- unusual bleeding from the sex organs
- flu-like symptoms with fever, aches and chills
- night sweats
- swelling of the lymph nodes
- unexplained weight loss
- persistent diarrhea
- unexplained fatigue

Many of these symptoms are the same as those of a cold, flu or other diseases. But people who have had sexual intercourse and who have any of these symptoms need to get an STD checkup. Those who engage in any risky behavior should get checked specifically for STD every time they have 1 of these symptoms and also when they have their regular health exams.

Some STD can be cured. Herpes, genital warts and HIV cannot. Early diagnosis is especially important in avoiding serious health consequences and disease transmission. Many STDs cause organ damage and other health problems. Chlamydia and gonorrhea can cause sterility in both men and women who do not get treated, by causing scar tissue to form that blocks the passages of the reproductive structures.

(continued...)

STD SYMPTOMS AND TREATMENT

STD can be passed from an infected mother to her child either before, during or after birth. Some pathogens pass through the placenta and into the fetus, while other STD pathogens are transmitted to the mucous membranes of the baby as it passes through the birth canal. HIV may be passed from a mother to her child during breastfeeding.

DIAGNOSIS AND TREATMENT

Having a specific set of symptoms is not sufficient for an accurate diagnosis; a variety of tests are used to identify the pathogens that cause different STDs. Some STDs are diagnosed by a blood test. A culture or microscopic examination of penile and vaginal discharge can identify other organisms that cause STD. Sometimes observation of symptoms, such as warts or fluid-filled blisters are all that is needed to make a diagnosis.

The disease must be correctly identified because the prescribed treatments are specific. For example, although the symptoms for gonorrhea and chlamydia are very similar, the diseases are commonly treated with 2 different types of antibiotic.

Treatment of incurable STD involves relieving the discomfort of the disease. Persons who have herpes can keep the blisters dry, soak in warm baths and take aspirin to relieve aches and fever. Some antiviral agents used as ointments and oral medications have been effective in reducing the frequency of herpes recurrences and the discomfort of the initial outbreak. Genital warts are removed by topical medications or surgery, cauterizing, freezing or vaporizing with a carbon dioxide laser.

Many agencies and organizations provide information, diagnosis and treatment related to STD. Every effort is made to make sure that diagnosis and treatment is confidential and provided at minimal or no cost. In most states, minors can obtain information, diagnosis and treatment without the knowledge or consent of parents.

(continued...)

STD Symptoms and Treatment

HOTLINES

A number of national hotlines offer information about STD. The CDC National AIDS Hotline can arrange a group call for your class. There is a limit of 15 minutes on calls and a speaker phone is required. Contact the CDC National AIDS Hotline for details (Attn: Classroom Call, P.O. Box 13827, Research Triangle Park, NC 27709).

National AIDS Hotline
(800) 342-2437
(800) 344-7432 (Spanish)
(800) 243-7889 (TTD/TTY)

Teen Hotline
(800) 440-TEEN
(open Friday and Saturday 6:00 p.m.–12:00 a.m. EST)

CDC National Clearinghouse
(800) 458-5231

World Health Organization
(202) 861-4346

National STD Hotline
(800) 227-8922

National Gay Task Force
AIDS Information Hotline
(800) 221-7044

San Francisco AIDS Foundation
(800) FOR-AIDS

Key

Read the case study and answer the questions.

Rosa and Ramon

1. Which STD might Rosa have? *herpes*
2. How can Rosa be cured? *There is no cure for herpes.*
3. What might happen if Rosa becomes pregnant? *She might transmit herpes to her baby.*

Melissa and Josh

1. What symptoms probably alerted Josh to his condition? *itching and burning around the sex organs; small, bumpy warts on and around the sex organs*
2. What might happen if Melissa and Josh have unprotected intercourse? *Melissa may get genital warts.*
3. Could Melissa get genital warts if Josh uses a condom and she uses nonoxynol-9? *Yes. Although preventive behavior helps prevent STD, only abstinence is 100% effective in preventing STD.*
4. What are the consequences of genital warts? *More warts can grow, precancerous conditions may develop, and the virus can be passed to a baby during childbirth.*

Frederick

1. Which STD does Frederick probably have? *syphilis*
2. Since the symptoms went away, is Frederick cured? *no*
3. What will the next symptoms probably be? *2nd stage symptoms—hair loss, flu-like symptoms, a rash on the body*
4. What will happen if Frederick does not get treated? *Frederick may transmit syphilis to his other sexual partner(s), develop heart disease, brain damage, blindness or may even die.*

Michael and Sunny

1. Which STD might Michael have? *HIV infection*
2. How could Michael have gotten this STD? *through unprotected sex or injection drug use*
3. What are the consequences of this STD for Michael, Sunny and their unborn child: *Michael may have transmitted HIV to his wife, Sunny, through sexual intercourse. If Sunny is infected with HIV, her unborn child may also become infected.*

UNDERSTANDING HIV

TIME

1 period

ACTIVITIES

1. Needing to Know About HIV

2. Answering Questions

UNDERSTANDING HIV

OBJECTIVE

Students will be able to:

> Summarize essential information about HIV infection and prevention.

GETTING STARTED

Have:

- posterboard, 6 pieces
- markers

Copy for each student:

- Dr. Know (8.1)

UNIT OVERVIEW

PURPOSE

Building on the understanding of STD developed in previous units, this lesson addresses specific information about HIV infection. Knowledge about HIV provides the basis for avoiding infection.

MAIN POINTS

* HIV infection is caused by a virus that affects the immune system.
* Many people with HIV infection have no symptoms; others are only occasionally ill.
* Persons with HIV infection who have a T-cell count below 200 are diagnosed as having AIDS.

REVIEW

To increase your understanding of HIV, review **About HIV** *Instant Expert* (p. 101) and **Dr. Know** *Key* (p. 104).

VOCABULARY

AIDS—Acquired Immune Deficiency Syndrome; a disease caused by a virus that damages the body's immune system.

helper T-cell—A specialized blood cell that helps direct the immune system's response to infection.

HIV—Human immunodeficiency virus; the virus that causes AIDS.

HIV-infected—Refers to a person with HIV, who may be without symptoms, have mild or severe symptoms, or have a diagnosis of AIDS.

immune system—The body's system of defense against disease.

1. NEEDING TO KNOW ABOUT HIV

25 minutes

❋

MATERIALS

◆ Dr. Know (8.1)

❋

COMMUNITY LINK

Invite someone with HIV or someone who works with people with HIV to speak to the class about what it's like to live with HIV infection.

This is a powerful way to help students personalize the importance of HIV prevention behavior. It is, however, an activity that must be approved locally. It is recommended that teachers, administrators, parents and community members work together to set up a speaker program that is appropriate for your community.

Brainstorm questions about HIV

Distribute the **Dr. Know** activity sheet and ask students to read the letter and the questions. Conduct a brainstorming session to identify additional questions students may have. List the additional questions on the board and have students add them to the list on the activity sheet.

Discuss HIV infection

Lead a class discussion on HIV infection, using the **About HIV** *Instant Expert* as a guide. Suggest that students write the answers to the questions on the **Dr. Know** activity sheet as they are discussed.

Dyads answer questions

Ask students to choose a partner and review their answers to the questions on the **Dr. Know** activity sheet, including the questions the class brainstormed.

Recap activity

Review the **Dr. Know** activity sheet questions and answers with the class. Clarify any misconceptions, using the **About HIV** *Instant Expert* as a guide.

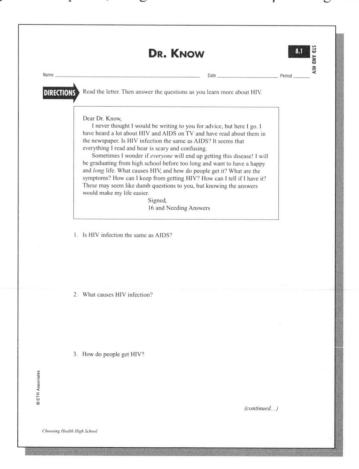

2. ANSWERING QUESTIONS

Groups create posters

Divide the class into 6 groups. Assign each group a question from the **Dr. Know** activity sheet, and distribute posterboard and markers. Explain the group assignment:

- Design a poster that presents information to answer the question.
- Be creative and use illustrations to present the information in an eye-catching manner.

Display posters

Provide an area in the classroom or the school to display students' posters.

25 minutes

MATERIALS

- Dr. Know (8.1)
- posterboard, 6 pieces
- markers

COMMUNITY LINK

Have students contact local community sites, such as libraries or stores, and ask permission to display their posters.

EVALUATION

REVIEW

♦ About HIV *Instant Expert*
(p. 101)

MATERIALS

♦ completed Dr. Know (8.1), from
Activity 1

♦ student posters, from Activity 2

OBJECTIVE

Students will be able to

> **Summarize essential information about HIV infection and prevention.**

Assess students' responses on the **Dr. Know** activity sheet and their work on the posters for their ability to summarize essential facts about HIV.

CRITERIA

Look for:

- accurate responses to questions
- portrayal of factual information about HIV
- presentation of prevention actions

About HIV

WHAT IS HIV INFECTION?

HIV infection is caused by the human immunodeficiency virus (HIV), sometimes called the AIDS virus. HIV infection affects people in a variety of ways. Some people who are infected do not have symptoms yet, some have mild symptoms, and some have severe symptoms. Many people with HIV infection look and feel well for years, but they can still pass the virus to others.

HIV attacks the helper T-cells of the immune system. This impairs the body's ability to fight serious infection, cancer and other illnesses. The virus can also affect the brain, causing a variety of problems with the nervous system.

Anyone infected with HIV has HIV infection. An AIDS diagnosis is given when a person with HIV infection has developed signs and symptoms of severe immune system impairment. Usually this is at an advanced stage of infection. Scientists do not know yet if everyone who is infected with HIV will eventually develop AIDS. The time period between infection with HIV and the development of AIDS can be as short as a few months or longer than a decade.

Some people think only certain members of "high-risk groups" get HIV infection. This is *not* true. Anyone who engages in risky behaviors can become infected with HIV.

HOW IS HIV TRANSMITTED?

HIV lives in certain body fluids, such as blood, semen and vaginal fluids. People become infected with HIV by taking the blood, semen or vaginal fluids of an infected person into their bodies. There are 3 ways this might happen:

- **Unprotected sexual intercourse.** People may take in the blood, semen or vaginal fluids of a sexual partner during vaginal, oral or anal intercourse. "Unprotected" intercourse means no condom or latex barrier was used.
- **Sharing needles or other equipment in injection drug use.** Injection drug users frequently share needles. Small amounts of blood may remain in a needle or syringe as it is passed from person to person. Sharing needles for other purposes (tattooing, ear or body piercing, injecting steroids or insulin) is also risky.
- **From an infected woman to her fetus or newborn.** A pregnant woman with HIV has an approximately 25% chance of passing the virus to her fetus or newborn. Medications taken during pregnancy and at the time of delivery can help protect the fetus from infection, though some risk of transmission remains. There are a few cases where a woman with HIV has transmitted the virus to her baby through her breast milk.

(continued...)

ABOUT HIV

In the early 1980s, a number of people were infected with HIV through blood transfusions, and people with hemophilia were infected through being treated with medicines manufactured from human blood. Today, medicines for hemophilia are manufactured so they cannot transmit HIV, and, since 1985, blood donated for transfusions has been tested for HIV.

People do **not** get HIV from casual, day-to-day contact with infected individuals.

IS THERE A CURE OR VACCINE FOR HIV?

Currently, there is neither a cure nor a vaccine to prevent HIV infection. Although millions of dollars have been spent to develop a cure or a vaccine, scientists say it will be years before either may become available.

WHAT ARE THE SYMPTOMS OF HIV?

For most people with HIV infection, the first symptoms occur about 2–6 weeks after infection with the virus. These symptoms may be so mild that the person thinks it is only a minor illness, such as flu. The symptoms include fever, sweating, fatigue, headache, swollen glands and a sore throat. At this stage, the symptoms pass without any treatment and may not recur for many years.

The next symptoms to appear are unexplained weight loss or fatigue, fever and night sweats, diarrhea, swollen glands, dry cough and white spots or unusual sores on the tongue or mouth. When these symptoms occur they either don't go away or keep coming back.

Once the helper T-cell count equals or falls below 200, the person is diagnosed as having AIDS. As the infected person's helper T-cells are destroyed, the immune system is not able to fight off "opportunistic infections," such as pneumonia and rare types of cancer that can cause death.

HOW CAN PEOPLE TELL IF THEY HAVE HIV?

When a person is infected with HIV, the body produces antibodies to the virus. Special blood tests can detect these HIV antibodies. If a person suspects that he or she has HIV infection, it is important to get tested. The test is the only way to know for sure. There is no known cure for HIV infection, but early treatment can delay the start of symptoms.

(continued...)

About HIV

HOW CAN PEOPLE PROTECT THEMSELVES FROM HIV?

- Do not have sexual intercourse (vaginal, oral or anal) with anyone—abstinence.
- Have sexual intercourse only with 1 uninfected, mutually faithful partner who does not use injection drugs or share needles with anyone—mutual monogamy.
- Use condoms or latex barriers for all forms of sexual intercourse. (This is not 100% safe, but significantly reduces HIV risk for people who are sexually active.)
- Do not use injection drugs.
- Never share needles, syringes or other equipment for injection drug use, injecting steroids or vitamins, ear or body piercing, tattooing or any other purpose.
- Avoid all blood-to-blood contact. Follow universal precautions for avoiding transmission of blood-borne diseases in first-aid situations.

DR. KNOW

KEY

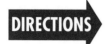

DIRECTIONS Read the letter. Then answer the questions as you learn more about HIV.

> Dear Dr. Know,
>
> I never thought I would be writing to you for advice, but here I go. I have heard a lot about HIV and AIDS on TV and have read about them in the newspaper. Is HIV infection the same as AIDS? It seems that everything I read and hear is scary and confusing.
>
> Sometimes I wonder if *everyone* will end up getting this disease! I will be graduating from high school before too long and want to have a happy and *long* life. What causes HIV, and how do people get it? What are the symptoms? How can I keep from getting HIV? How can I tell if I have it? These may seem like dumb questions to you, but knowing the answers would make my life easier.
>
> Signed,
> 16 and Needing Answers

1. Is HIV infection the same as AIDS?

   No. Everyone who is infected with HIV has HIV infection. To be diagnosed with AIDS, an HIV-infected person must have a helper T-cell count below 200.

2. What causes HIV infection?

   HIV infection is caused when the human immunodeficiency virus (HIV) gets into a person's body. HIV lives in certain body fluids. It can be transmitted in semen, blood or vaginal fluids.

3. How do people get HIV?

   People can get HIV in 3 ways: (1) sexual intercourse (vaginal, oral or anal) with an infected person; (2) sharing needles or syringes with an infected person; or (3) from infected, pregnant mothers to their babies before or during birth or after birth through breastfeeding.

   (continued...)

Dr. Know

Key, Continued

4. What are the symptoms of HIV infection?

    Most people have no symptoms or very mild symptoms at first. They may experience flu-like symptoms, such as sore throat, fever and headache. Later, a person with HIV may have unexplained weight loss, swollen glands, fever and night sweats, diarrhea, dry cough and unusual sores in the mouth. When the individual's immune system gets very weak, other diseases such as rare cancers and pneumonia can affect the body.

5. How can I tell if I have HIV?

    A test that detects whether blood contains antibodies to HIV is the only sure way to tell if a person is infected with HIV.

6. How can I protect myself from HIV?

    The best ways to avoid HIV infection are to practice sexual abstinence or mutual monogamy with 1 uninfected, mutually faithful partner, and not to use injection drugs or share needles and syringes for any purpose. A behavior that is not 100% effective but that reduces the risk of getting HIV is the correct use of latex condoms and barriers during sexual intercourse.

FINAL EVALUATION

FINAL EVALUATION

Groups design plans

Divide the class into groups of 4. Distribute butcher paper and markers. Tell groups they are to take the role of a group of teachers designing an educational program for high school students to prevent STD and HIV infection.

Explain the group assignment:

- Identify the goals of your program.
- Describe the important information needed by students.
- Identify the important skills needed by students.
- Design a way to present the information and skills to high school students.
- Prepare to present your plan to the class.

Groups present plans

Have groups report their plans to the class. Ask groups to explain why they felt particular information and skills were important to include. Allow time for class discussion.

CRITERIA

Assess group presentations to evaluate students' knowledge about STD and ways to prevent infection and their ability to identify and demonstrate communication, decision-making and assertiveness skills regarding sexual choices. Look for:

- Complete descriptions of methods of transmission for various STDs, including HIV.
- Accurate descriptions of effective methods of protection from STD, including HIV.
- Specific examples of communication, decision-making and assertiveness skills that can be used in preventing STD and HIV infection.

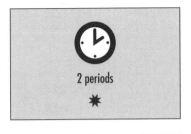

2 periods

MATERIALS

- butcher paper
- markers

APPENDIXES

Why Comprehensive School Health?

Components of a
Comprehensive Health Program

The Teacher's Role

Teaching Strategies

Glossary

References

WHY COMPREHENSIVE SCHOOL HEALTH?

The quality of life we ultimately achieve is determined in large part by the health decisions we make, the subsequent behaviors we adopt, and the public policies that promote and support the establishment of healthy behaviors.

A healthy student is capable of growing and learning; of producing new knowledge and ideas; of sharing, interacting and living peacefully with others in a complex and changing society. Fostering healthy children is the shared responsibility of families, communities and schools.

Health behaviors, the most important predictors of current and future health status, are influenced by a variety of factors. Factors that lead to and support the establishment of healthy behaviors include:

- awareness and knowledge of health issues
- the skills necessary to practice healthy behaviors
- opportunities to practice healthy behaviors
- support and reinforcement for the practice of healthy behaviors

The perception that a particular healthy behavior is worthwhile often results in young people becoming advocates, encouraging others to adopt the healthy behavior. When these young advocates exert pressure on peers to adopt healthy behaviors, a healthy social norm is established (e.g., tobacco use is unacceptable in this school).

Because health behaviors are learned, they can be shaped and changed. Partnerships between family members, community leaders, teachers and school leaders are a vital key to the initial development and maintenance of children's healthy behaviors and can also play a role in the modification of unhealthy behaviors. Schools, perhaps more than any other single agency in our society, have the opportunity to influence factors that shape the future health and productivity of Americans.

When young people receive reinforcement for the practice of a healthy behavior, they feel good about the healthy behavior. Reinforcement and the subsequent good feeling increase the likelihood that an individual will continue to practice a behavior and thereby establish a positive health habit. The good feeling and the experience of success motivate young people to place a high value on the behavior (e.g., being a nonsmoker is good).

From *Step by Step to Comprehensive School Health,* W. M. Kane (Santa Cruz, CA: ETR Associates, 1992).

COMPONENTS OF A COMPREHENSIVE HEALTH PROGRAM

The school's role in fostering the development of healthy students involves more than providing classes in health. There are 8 components of a comprehensive health education program:

- **School Health Instruction**—Instruction is the in-class aspect of the program. As in other subject areas, a scope of content defines the field. Application of classroom instruction to real life situations is critical.

- **Healthy School Environment**—The school environment includes both the physical and psychological surroundings of students, faculty and staff. The physical environment should be free of hazards; the psychological environment should foster healthy development.

- **School Health Services**—School health services offer a variety of activities that address the health status of students and staff.

- **Physical Education and Fitness**—Participation in physical education and fitness activities promotes healthy development. Students need information about how and why to be active and encouragement to develop skills that will contribute to fitness throughout their lives.

- **School Nutrition and Food Services**—The school's nutritional program provides an excellent opportunity to model healthy behaviors. Schools that provide healthy food choices and discourage availability of unhealthy foods send a clear message to students about the importance of good nutrition.

- **School-Based Counseling and Personal Support**—School counseling and support services play an important role in responding to special needs and providing personal support for individual students, teachers and staff. These services can also provide programs that promote schoolwide mental, emotional and social well-being.

- **Schoolsite Health Promotion**—Health promotion is a combination of educational, organizational and environmental activities designed to encourage students and staff to adopt healthier lifestyles and become better consumers of health care services. It views the school and its activities as a total environment.

- **School, Family and Community Health Promotion Partnerships**—Partnerships that unite schools, families and communities can address communitywide issues. These collaborative partnerships are the cornerstone of health promotion and disease prevention.

THE TEACHER'S ROLE

The teacher plays a critical role in meeting the challenge to empower students with the knowledge, skills and ability to make healthy behavior choices throughout their lives.

Instruction

Teachers need to provide students with learning opportunities that go beyond knowledge. Instruction must include the chance to practice skills that will help students make healthy decisions.

Involve Families and Communities

The issues in health are real-life issues, issues that families and communities deal with daily. Students need to see the relationship of what they learn at school to what occurs in their homes and their communities.

Model Healthy Behavior

Teachers educate students by their actions too. Students watch the way teachers manage health issues in their own lives. Teachers need to ask themselves if they are modeling the health behaviors they want students to adopt.

Maintain a Healthy Environment

The classroom environment has both physical and emotional aspects. It is the teacher's role to maintain a safe physical environment. It is also critical to provide an environment that is sensitive, respectful and developmentally appropriate.

Establish Groundrules

It is very important to establish classroom groundrules before discussing sensitive topics or issues. Setting and consistently enforcing groundrules establishes an atmosphere of respect, in which students can share and explore their personal thoughts, feelings, opinions and values.

Refer Students to Appropriate Services

Teachers may be the first to notice illness, learning disorders or emotional distress in students. The role of the teacher is one of referral. Most districts have guidelines for teachers to follow.

Legal Compliance

Teachers must make every effort to communicate to parents and other family members about the nature of the curriculum. Instruction about certain topics, such as sexuality, HIV or drug use, often must follow notification guidelines regulated by state law. Most states also require teachers to report any suspected cases of child abuse or neglect.

TEACHING STRATEGIES

The resource books incorporate a variety of instructional strategies. This variety is essential in addressing the needs of different kinds of learners. Different strategies are grouped according to their general education purpose. When sequenced, these strategies are designed to help students acquire the knowledge and skills they need to choose healthy behavior. Strategies are identified with each activity. Some strategies are traditional, while others are more interactive, encouraging students to help each other learn.

The strategies are divided into 4 categories according to their general purpose:

- providing key information
- encouraging creative expression
- sharing thoughts, feelings and opinions
- developing critical thinking

The following list details strategies in each category.

Providing Key Information

Information provides the foundation for learning. Before students can move to higher-level thinking, they need to have information about a topic. In lieu of a textbook, this series uses a variety of strategies to provide students the information they need to take actions for their health.

Anonymous Question Box

An anonymous question box provides the opportunity for all students to get answers to questions they might be hesitant to ask in class. It also gives teachers time to think about answers to difficult questions or to look for more information.

Questions should be reviewed and responded to regularly, and all questions placed in the box should be taken seriously. If you don't know the answer to a question, research it and report back to students.

You may feel that some questions would be better answered privately. Offer students the option of signing their questions if they want a private, written answer. Any questions not answered in class can then be answered privately.

Current Events

Analyzing local, state, national and international current events helps students relate classroom discussion to everyday life. It also helps students understand how local, national and global events and policies affect health status. Resources for current

TEACHING STRATEGIES

events include newspapers, magazines and other periodicals, radio and television programs and news.

Demonstrations and Experiments

Teachers, guest speakers or students can use demonstrations and experiments to show how something works or why something is important. These activities also provide a way to show the correct process for doing something, such as a first-aid procedure.

Demonstrations and experiments should be carefully planned and conducted. They often involve the use of supporting materials.

Games and Puzzles

Games and puzzles can be used to provide a different environment in which learning can take place. They are frequently amusing and sometimes competitive.

Many types of games and puzzles can be adapted to present and review health concepts. It may be a simple question-and-answer game or an adaptation of games such as Bingo, Concentration or Jeopardy. Puzzles include crosswords and word searches.

A game is played according to a specific set of rules. Game rules should be clear and simple. Using groups of students in teams rather than individual contestants helps involve the entire class.

Guest Speakers

Guest speakers can be recruited from students' families, the school and the community. They provide a valuable link between the classroom and the "real world."

Speakers should be screened before being invited to present to the class. They should have some awareness of the level of student knowledge and should be given direction for the content and focus of the presentation.

Interviewing

Students can interview experts and others about a specific topic either inside or outside of class. Invite experts, family members and others to visit class, or ask students to interview others (family members or friends) outside of class.

Advance preparation for an organized interview session increases the learning potential. A brainstorming session before the interview allows students to develop questions to ask during the interview.

TEACHING STRATEGIES

Oral Presentations

Individual students or groups or panels of students can present information orally to the rest of the class. Such presentations may sometimes involve the use of charts or posters to augment the presentation.

Students enjoy learning and hearing from each other, and the experience stimulates positive interaction. It also helps build students' communication skills.

Encouraging Creative Expression

Student creativity should be encouraged and challenged. Creative expression provides the opportunity to integrate language arts, fine arts and personal experience into a lesson. It also helps meet the diverse needs of students with different learning styles.

Artistic Expression or Creative Writing

Students may be offered a choice of expressing themselves in art or through writing. They may write short stories, poems or letters, or create pictures or collages about topics they are studying. Such a choice accommodates the differing needs and talents of students.

This technique can be used as a follow-up to most lessons. Completed work should be displayed in the classroom, at school or in the community.

Dramatic Presentations

Dramatic presentations may take the form of skits or mock news, radio or television shows. They can be presented to the class or to larger groups in the school or community. When equipment is available, videotapes of these presentations provide an opportunity to present students' work to other classes in the school and other groups in the community.

Such presentations are highly motivating activities, because they actively involve students in learning desired concepts. They also allow students to practice new behaviors in a safe setting and help them personalize information presented in class.

Roleplays

Acting out difficult situations provides students practice in new behaviors in a safe setting. Sometimes students are given a part to play, and other times they are given an idea and asked to improvise. Students need time to decide the central action of the situation and how they will resolve it before they make their presentation. Such activities are highly motivating because they actively involve students in learning desired concepts or practicing certain behaviors.

Sharing Thoughts, Feelings and Opinions

In the sensitive areas of health education, students may have a variety of opinions and feelings. Providing a safe atmosphere in which to discuss opinions and feelings encourages students to share their ideas and listen and learn from others. Such discussion also provides an opportunity to clarify misinformation and correct misconceptions.

Brainstorming

Brainstorming is used to stimulate discussion of an issue or topic. It can be done with the whole class or in smaller groups. It can be used both to gather information and to share thoughts and opinions.

All statements should be accepted without comment or judgment from the teacher or other students. Ideas can be listed on the board, on butcher paper or newsprint or on a transparency. Brainstorming should continue until all ideas have been exhausted or a predetermined time limit has been reached.

Class Discussion

A class discussion led by the teacher or by students is a valuable educational strategy. It can be used to initiate, amplify or summarize a lesson. Such discussions also provide a way to share ideas, opinions and concerns that may have been generated in small group work.

Clustering

Clustering is a simple visual technique that involves diagraming ideas around a main topic. The main topic is written on the board and circled. Other related ideas are then attached to the central idea or to each other with connecting lines.

Clustering can be used as an adjunct to brainstorming. Because there is no predetermined number of secondary ideas, clustering can accommodate all brainstorming ideas.

Continuum Voting

Continuum voting is a stimulating discussion technique. Students express the extent to which they agree or disagree with a statement read by the teacher. The classroom

TEACHING STRATEGIES

should be prepared for this activity with a sign that says "Agree" on one wall and a sign that says "Disagree" on the opposite wall. There should be room for students to move freely between the 2 signs.

As the teacher reads a statement, students move to a point between the signs that reflects their thoughts or feelings. The closer to the "Agree" sign they stand, the stronger their agreement. The closer to the "Disagree" sign they stand, the stronger their disagreement. A position in the center between the signs indicates a neutral stance.

Dyad Discussion

Working in pairs allows students to provide encouragement and support to each other. Students who may feel uncomfortable sharing in the full class may be more willing to share their thoughts and feelings with 1 other person. Depending on the task, dyads may be temporary, or students may meet regularly with a partner and work together to achieve their goals.

Forced Field Analysis

This strategy is used to discuss an issue that is open to debate. Students analyze a situation likely to be approved by some students and opposed by others. For example, if the subject of discussion was the American diet, some students might support the notion that Americans consume healthy foods because of the wide variety of foods available. Other students might express concern about the amount of foods that are high in sodium, fat and sugar.

Questioning skills are critical to the success of this technique. A good way to open such a discussion is to ask students, "What questions should you ask to determine if you support or oppose this idea?" The pros and cons of students' analysis can be charted on the board or on a transparency.

Journal Writing

Journal writing affords the opportunity for thinking and writing. Expressive writing requires that students become actively involved in the learning process. However, writing may become a less effective tool for learning if students must worry about spelling and punctuation. Students should be encouraged to write freely in their journals, without fear of evaluation.

Panel Discussion

Panel discussions provide an opportunity to discuss different points of view about a health topic, problem or issue. Students can research and develop supporting

Teaching Strategies

arguments for different sides. Such research and discussion enhances understanding of content.

Panel members may include experts from the community as well as students. Panel discussions are usually directed by a moderator and may be followed by a question and answer period.

Self-Assessment

Personal inventories provide a tool for self-assessment. Providing privacy around personal assessments allows students to be honest in their responses. Volunteers can share answers or the questions can be discussed in general, but no students should have to share answers they would prefer to keep private. Students can use the information to set personal goals for changing behaviors.

Small Groups

Students working together can help stimulate each other's creativity. Small group activities are cooperative, but have less formal structure than cooperative learning groups. These activities encourage collective thinking and provide opportunities for students to work with others and increase social skills.

Surveys and Inventories

Surveys and inventories can be used to assess knowledge, attitudes, beliefs and practices. These instruments can be used to gather knowledge about a variety of groups, including students, parents and other family members, and teachers.

Students can use surveys others have designed or design their own. When computers are available, students can use them to summarize their information, create graphs and prepare presentations of the data.

Developing Critical Thinking

Critical thinking skills help students analyze health topics and issues. These activities require that students learn to gather information, consider the consequences of actions and behaviors and make responsible decisions. They challenge students to perform higher-level thinking and clearly communicate their ideas.

Case Studies

Case studies provide written histories of a problem or situation. Students can read, discuss and analyze these situations. This strategy encourages student involvement and helps students personalize the health-related concepts presented in class.

TEACHING STRATEGIES

Cooperative Learning Groups

Cooperative learning is an effective teaching strategy that has been shown to have a positive effect on students' achievement and interpersonal skills. Students can work in small groups to disseminate and share information, analyze ideas or solve problems. The size of the group depends on the nature of the lesson and the make-up of the class. Groups work best with from 2–6 members.

Group structure will affect the success of the lessons. Groups can be formed by student choice, random selection, or a more formal, teacher-influenced process. Groups seem to function best when they represent the variety and balance found in the classroom. Groups also work better when each student has a responsibility within the group (reader, recorder, timer, reporter, etc.).

While groups are working on their tasks, the teacher should move from group to group, answering questions and dealing with any problems that arise. At the conclusion of the group process, some closure should take place.

Debates

Students can debate the pros and cons of many issues relating to health. Suggesting that students defend an opposing point of view provides an additional learning experience.

During a debate, each side has the opportunity to present their arguments and to refute each others' arguments. After the debate, class members can choose the side with which they agree.

Factual Writing

Once students have been presented with information about a topic, a variety of writing assignments can challenge them to clarify and express their ideas and opinions. Position papers, letters to the editor, proposals and public service announcements provide a forum in which students can express their opinions, supporting them with facts, figures and reasons.

Media Analysis

Students can analyze materials from a variety of media, including printed matter, music, TV programs, movies, video games and advertisements, to identify health-related messages. Such analysis might include identifying the purpose of the piece, the target audience, underlying messages, motivations and stereotypes.

TEACHING STRATEGIES

Personal Contracts

Personal contracts, individual commitments to changing behavior, can help students make positive changes in their health-related behaviors. The wording of a personal contract may include the behavior to be changed, a plan for changing the behavior and the identification of possible problems and support systems.

However, personal contracts should be used with caution. Behavior change may be difficult, especially in the short term. Students should be encouraged to make personal contracts around goals they are likely to meet.

Research

Research requires students to seek information to complete a task. Students may be given prepared materials that they must use to complete an assignment, or they may have to locate resources and gather information on their own. As part of this strategy, students must compile and organize the information they collect.

GLOSSARY

A

abstinence—Avoiding sexual intercourse.

ad-lib—To speak spontaneously, not in a prepared script.

AIDS—Acquired Immune Deficiency Syndrome; a disease caused by a virus that damages the body's immune system, making the infected person susceptible to a wide range of serious diseases.

antibiotics—Drugs derived from molds and fungi; used mainly to treat bacterial infection.

antibody—A protein produced by the body's white blood cells to neutralize or destroy invading foreign chemical substances.

antigens—Components of bacteria and viruses that cause the immune system to react when they enter the body.

B

bacteria—One-cell microscopic organisms found in living things, air, soil and water; some are beneficial to humans, some cause disease.

blood—Fluid circulating through the heart, arteries and veins.

bloodstream—The blood flowing through the body.

blood transfusion—The transfer of blood from a donor into the veins of another person to treat illness or injury.

body fluids—Any of the fluids produced by the body: tears, mucous, saliva, sweat, vaginal secretions, semen, blood or urine. HIV can be found in any of these fluids but is only transmissible through blood, semen and vaginal fluids.

body language—A form of nonverbal communication made up of facial expressions, body movement, posture, gestures, etc., that are clues to a person's thoughts and feelings. Sometimes body language can speak louder than words.

C

casual contact—Day-to-day contact between people at home, school, work or in the community, which does not involve sexual interaction or the sharing of needles.

***caution* situation**—A circumstance that signals the approach of a *danger* situation.

chlamydia—Any of several common, often asymptomatic, sexually transmitted diseases, caused by bacteria, that infect the reproductive organs.

communicable disease—A disease that is spread from person to person either directly or indirectly.

condom—A protective device used to cover the penis or vagina and cervix during intercourse to prevent pregnancy and the transmission of disease. Latex condoms are effective in helping prevent transmission of HIV.

confidential—Secret or private.

contagious—Able to pass a communicable disease to another person by direct or indirect contact, depending on the disease.

contraception—The use of devices or chemicals to prevent pregnancy.

D

danger **situation**—A circumstance that may lead to sexual intercourse unless immediate action is taken.

decision—The result of making up one's mind; a judgment or conclusion.

decision making—Making choices; using one's judgment.

disease—A particular destructive process in an organ or organism, with a specific cause and characteristic symptoms; an illness.

disease prevention—Steps taken to help prevent the negative effects of disease.

E

effect—Something brought about by a cause or an agent; a result or consequence.

ejaculation—The expulsion of semen from the penis.

expose—To come in contact with an influence, such as a disease or other risk.

F

female condom—A polyurethane pouch inserted into the vagina to prevent the exchange of body fluids during intercourse.

G

genital warts—A sexually transmitted disease caused by the *human papilloma virus*; causes small, bumpy warts on and around the sex organs or anus.

gonorrhea—One of the most common sexually transmitted diseases, caused by bacteria and transmitted by direct contact, usually of a sexual nature; can cause sterility.

H

health—The general condition of the body.

helper T-cell—A specialized blood cell that helps direct the immune system's response to infection.

herpes—An STD, caused by virus, that results in painful blisters and flu-like symptoms.

herpes simplex—A virus associated with sores either around the mouth and lips or on the genitals.

HIV—Human immunodeficiency virus; the virus that causes AIDS.

GLOSSARY

HIV-infected—Refers to a person with HIV, who may be without symptoms of immune suppression, may have mild or severe symptoms, or may have a diagnosis of AIDS.

hospice—A concept of care for the terminally ill that provides supportive care in a homelike environment.

I

immune system—The body's system of defense against disease; consists of specialized cells and proteins in the blood and other body fluids.

immunity—The state of being able to resist a particular disease by counteracting the potential effects of a foreign substance or disease-causing microorganism.

infection—The establishment of a pathogen in a susceptible host.

infectious agent—A microorganism that causes disease (e.g., bacterium, virus or fungi).

intercourse—A type of sexual contact involving one of the following: (1) insertion of a man's penis into a woman's vagina (vaginal intercourse), (2) placement of the mouth on the genitals of another person (oral intercourse), or (3) insertion of a man's penis into the anus of another person (anal intercourse).

L

latex barrier—A rectangular piece of latex used to cover the vulva during oral intercourse.

M

male condom—A sheath stretched over the penis to prevent the exchange of body fluids during intercourse.

monogamy—Having only 1 sex partner.

mucous membranes—Tissues that line body openings.

myth—Popular fable or folk tale; a fiction or half-truth.

N

NGU—Nongonococcal urethritis; a sexually transmitted disease caused by bacteria; symptoms are similar to gonorrhea.

nonoxynol-9—A chemical that kills sperm and may help protect against the pathogens that cause some STD; can be used as a lubricant to increase condom effectiveness.

no-risk behavior—Action that does not transmit STD.

GLOSSARY

O

opinion—A conclusion or judgment held with confidence, but falling short of positive knowledge.

opportunistic infection—An illness that does not normally affect healthy people but becomes a problem when the immune system is damaged.

P

pathogen—A microorganism that can cause disease; a specific agent that causes disease (e.g., a bacterium or virus).

perinatal—Pertaining to or occurring in the period surrounding birth; shortly before, during or shortly after birth.

perinatal transmission—Passing of an infection from a woman to her baby during birth.

***Pneumocystis carinii* pneumonia (PCP)**—The most common life-threatening opportunistic infection diagnosed in AIDS. Caused by a protozoan parasite, it causes difficulty in breathing and is the most common cause of death for people with AIDS.

prenatal transmission—Passing of an infection from a woman to her fetus before birth.

prevention—Hindering something from happening or existing, as in the case of disease.

protection behavior—Action that provides some protection against STD, or action that reduces the risk of spreading STD.

pubic lice—Parasites (tiny insects) that live in pubic hair, armpits or eyebrows and cause itching; transmitted by close physical contact with another person who has pubic lice, or by using clothing or bedding of such a person.

R

refusal—Saying no.

refusal skills—Ways to say no clearly and effectively while maintaining a relationship.

relationship building—Letting another person know one values the connection or relationship.

risk—The likelihood of injury, damage or other negative consequences following an action.

risky behavior—Action that may transmit STD; behavior that causes an increased likelihood of injury, damage or other negative consequences.

GLOSSARY

S

safer sex—Sexual activity that reduces the risk of HIV infection because no body fluids are exchanged.

saliva—A body fluid secreted into the mouth by salivary glands; may include traces of HIV in an infected person, but not enough to infect another.

semen—Thick, whitish fluid secreted from the penis during sexual orgasm; contains sperm.

sexual intercourse—Vaginal, oral or anal sex.

sexually transmitted disease (STD)—Any of a number of infectious diseases that are most commonly spread through sexual contact.

spermicide—Any substance used to help prevent pregnancy because of its ability to kill sperm.

sterile—Unable to have a child.

symptoms—Subjective evidence of disease; indications of the presence of a bodily disorder.

syphilis—A sexually transmitted disease, caused by bacteria, that results in open sores, skin rash, hair loss and damage to internal organs.

syringe—A device used to inject fluids into or withdraw them from something; some drugs are injected using a syringe.

T

transmission—The passing of infection from 1 person to another.

transmit—To pass infection from 1 person to another.

treatment—Care to reduce symptoms, cure a disease or change a condition.

V

vaccine—A preparation containing killed or weakened virus; administered to produce immunity to a specific disease organism or toxin.

vaginal fluids—Natural lubrication or secretions of the vagina, including those produced during periods of sexual arousal.

venereal disease (VD)—Another name for sexually transmitted disease.

virus—An organism formed of genetic material surrounded by a protein coating; technically, not a living organism since it cannot reproduce itself but must invade a living cell to replicate.

vulva—External female genitalia.

W

white blood cell—Any of the body's colorless blood cells; many different white blood cells help defend the body against infection as part of the immune system.

REFERENCES

Althaus, F. S. 1991. An ounce of prevention…STDs and women's health. *Family Planning Perspectives* 23:173–177.

Aral, S. O., and K. K. Holmes. 1991. Sexually transmitted diseases in the AIDS era. *Scientific American* 264:62–69.

Centers for Disease Control and Prevention. 1992, July. *HIV/AIDS surveillance report*. Atlanta, GA: U.S. Department of Health and Human Services.

Centers for Disease Control and Prevention. 1995, March. Youth risk behavior surveillance—United States, 1993. *Morbidity and Mortality Weekly Report* 44 (SS-1).

Cox, F. D. 1992. *The AIDS booklet*. 2d ed. Dubuque, IA: William C. Brown.

Hansen, W. B., B. L. Hahn and B. H. Wolkenstein. 1990. Perceived personal immunity: Beliefs and susceptibility to AIDS. *Journal of Sex Research* 28:99–123.

Herpes Resource Center. 1991. *Understanding herpes*. Research Triangle Park, NC: American Social Health Association.

Maticka-Tyndale, E. 1991. Sexual scripts and AIDS prevention variations in adherence to safer-sex guidelines by heterosexual adolescents. *Journal of Sex Research* 18:3–27.

Murphy, R. L. 1992. Sexually transmitted diseases. In *The biological and clinical basis of infectious diseases*, 4th ed., ed. S. T. Shulman, J. P. Phair and H. M. Sommers. Philadelphia, PA: W. B. Saunders.

Protecting your partner/relationship. 1992. *HPV News* 2 (2): 6.

Reitmeijer, C., J. Krebs, P. Feorino and F. Judson. 1988. Condoms as physical and chemical barriers against human immunodeficiency virus. *Journal of the American Medical Association* 259:1851–1853.

Schwebke, J. R. 1991a. Gonorrhea in the 90s. *Medical Aspects of Human Sexuality* 29:42–46.

Schwebke, J. R. 1991b. Syphilis in the 90s. *Medical Aspects of Human Sexuality* 29:44–49.

Stein, A. P. 1991. The chlamydia epidemic: Teenagers at risk. *Medical Aspects of Human Sexuality* 29:26–33.

MASTERS

CONTENTS

chlamydia

genital warts

gonorrhea

herpes

HIV infection

syphilis

- ## Sexual Intercourse (oral, vaginal or anal)

- ## Blood-to-Blood Contact

- ## Infected Women to Their Babies

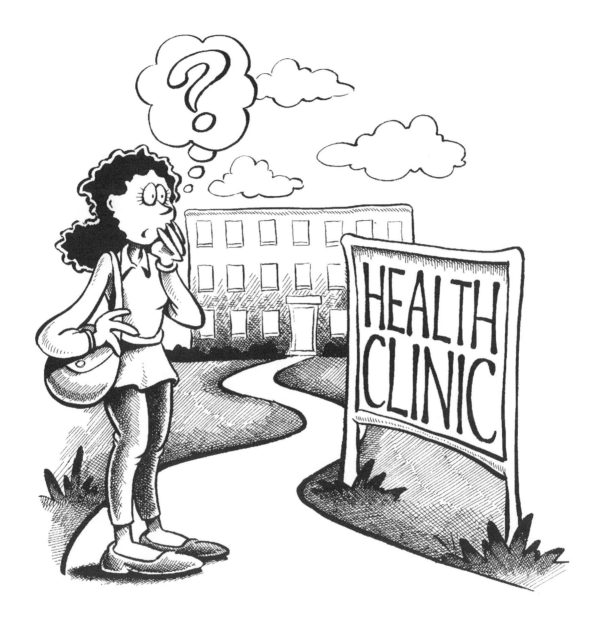

If you think you have an STD, get an STD checkup.

- **abstain from sexual intercourse**

- **don't use or share needles**

- **have only 1 mutually faithful, *uninfected* sexual partner**

- **get tested for STD before having sexual intercourse**

- **use a latex condom**

- **look for signs of STD**

- **use products with nonoxynol-9**

- **avoid alcohol and other drugs**

MAIN POINTS ABOUT STD

Name _____ Date _____ Period _____

COMMON STDs

chlamydia

genital warts

gonorrhea

herpes

HIV infection

syphilis

© ETR Associates

Choosing Health High School

STD IS SPREAD BY...

- **Sexual Intercourse**
  (oral, vaginal or anal)

- **Blood-to-Blood**
  Contact

- **Infected Women**
  to Their Babies

© ETR Associates

Choosing Health High School

WHAT DO YOU DO?

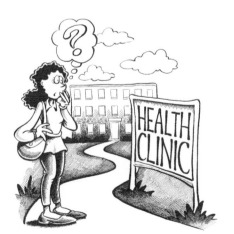

**If you think you have an STD,
get an STD checkup.**

© ETR Associates

Choosing Health High School

STD PREVENTION

- **abstain from sexual intercourse**

- **don't use or share needles**

- **have only 1 mutually faithful,
  uninfected sexual partner**

- **get tested for STD before
  having sexual intercourse**

- **use a latex condom**

- **look for signs of STD**

- **use products with nonoxynol-9**

- **avoid alcohol and other drugs**

© ETR Associates

Choosing Health High School

STD Facts

Name _____   Date _____ Period _____

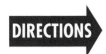 **DIRECTIONS** Answer the following questions.

1. What are sexually transmitted diseases (STDs)?

2. Name 6 of the most common STDs.

3. List 3 ways STD is spread.

4. How can you avoid getting an STD?

5. What advice would you give someone who thought he or she might have an STD?

6. Choose the best answer.
   Your risk of getting an STD is determined by:
   a. sexual orientation
   b. where you live
   c. poor nutrition
   d. your behavior
   e. your race

Comprehensive Health for High School

Name _____ Date _____ Period _____

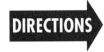 **DIRECTIONS** When the teacher says, "Select a partner," find the person who has M2 on his or her sheet. Shake hands with this person and write down his or her name. You will shake hands ONLY with M2 for the entire activity.

M1

fold here

Name

Partner 1–5 _____

Name _____ Date _____ Period _____

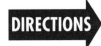 **DIRECTIONS** When the teacher says, "Select a partner," find the person who has M1 on his or her sheet. Shake hands with this person and write down his or her name. You will shake hands ONLY with M1 for the entire activity.

M2

fold here

- -

Name

Partner 1–5 _____

Name _____ Date _____ Period _____

DIRECTIONS When the teacher says, "Select a partner," put the glove on your hand. Leave the glove on for the entire activity. Shake hands with a new partner during each round and write down each partner's name.

C

fold here

- -

Names

Partner 1 _____

Partner 2 _____

Partner 3 _____

Partner 4 _____

Partner 5 _____

PASS IT AROUND—P?

Name _____ Date _____ Period _____

 When the teacher says, "Select a partner," put the glove on your hand. Leave the glove on for the first 2 handshakes. Take it off for the last 3 handshakes. Shake hands with a new partner during each round and write down each partner's name.

P?

fold here

- -

Names

Partner 1 _____

Partner 2 _____

Partner 3 _____

Partner 4 _____

Partner 5 _____

Name _____ Date _____ Period _____

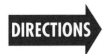 Do not shake hands with anyone.

A

fold here

- -

Names

Partner 1 *none* _____

Partner 2 *none* _____

Partner 3 *none* _____

Partner 4 *none* _____

Partner 5 *none* _____

Name _____ Date _____ Period _____

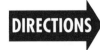 **DIRECTIONS** Shake hands with a new partner during each round and write down each partner's name.

I

fold here

- -

Names

Partner 1 _____

Partner 2 _____

Partner 3 _____

Partner 4 _____

Partner 5 _____

PASS IT AROUND

Name _____ Date _____ Period _____

 Shake hands with a new partner during each round and write down each partner's name.

- *fold here* -

Names

Partner 1 _____

Partner 2 _____

Partner 3 _____

Partner 4 _____

Partner 5 _____

NO RISK—PROTECTION—RISKY

Name _____ Date _____ Period _____

DIRECTIONS ▶ Put the behaviors listed at the bottom of the page in the correct category.

NO RISK

PROTECTION

RISKY

- vaginal intercourse with someone who uses injection drugs
- not injecting drugs
- abstinence
- oral intercourse using a condom or latex barrier
- sharing drug needles and syringes
- oral intercourse with multiple partners
- intercourse only with 1 mutually faithful, uninfected partner

- unprotected vaginal, oral or anal intercourse
- vaginal intercourse with someone you don't know well
- vaginal intercourse using a latex condom
- kissing
- body massage
- anal intercourse
- hugging

ABOUT ABSTINENCE

Name _____ Date _____ Period _____

DIRECTIONS ▶ *Directions:* Read about the 2 people in each scenario and decide which person you are most like. Mark an "X" anywhere along the line between the 2 names. You may feel exactly like one of these people, or you may have feelings somewhere in between.

1. Dominique believes that people should have intercourse if they are attracted to one another. She says that people should enjoy their bodies and express their sexual feelings openly.

   Jessica says that only people who are married to each other should have intercourse. She would not consider having sex with anyone unless he was her husband.

   Dominique   Jessica
   └──┘

2. Marcus says that anyone who has intercourse is asking for an STD. He believes that the only way to be safe is to practice abstinence.

   Jerome has unprotected intercourse but doesn't feel he is at risk for getting an STD. He thinks abstinence is unrealistic for teens.

   Marcus   Jerome
   └──┘

3. Ashley wants to finish school and get a good-paying job. She feels that getting pregnant or an STD would ruin her plans and her future. Sexual intercourse is out of the question for her right now. She doesn't want to take any chances with her future.

   Amber has several friends who already have babies and thinks that being a mother would be cool. Amber can't wait to meet someone she likes enough to have his baby.

   Ashley   Amber
   └──┘

4. Jason says the only way to really show someone you love them is to have sex with them. He feels that if someone doesn't care enough about him to have sex, he'll find someone who does. Jason says that STD only happens to people who live in big cities or shoot drugs.

   Jamal believes that waiting to have sex is a good way to show how much you care about a person. He says that talking and doing a lot of different things with that person is the best way to get close. Jamal doesn't worry about STD because he chooses to be abstinent.

   Jason   Jamal
   └──┘

Choosing Health High School

REASONS FOR CHOOSING ABSTINENCE

Name _____ Date _____ Period _____

 DIRECTIONS Read the 4 reasons for choosing abstinence and rank them in order of their importance to you (1 = most important, 2 = next important, 3 = third in importance, 4 = fourth in importance).

_____ religious or other personal reasons

_____ to prevent STD

_____ to prevent pregnancy

_____ for emotional protection

Choosing Health High School

Name _____ Date _____ Period _____

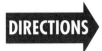 Use the steps to help you think through the choice about abstinence that the character in the case study has to make. Fill in each step.

A. State the problem.

B. List the options.
   1. _____
   2. _____

C. List the consequences for each option.
   Option 1 _____
   1. _____
   2. _____
   3. _____
   4. _____
   5. _____

   Option 2 _____
   1. _____
   2. _____
   3. _____
   4. _____
   5. _____

D. Make the choice.

E. Evaluate the choice.

DECISION-MAKING PRACTICE

DIRECTIONS Cut apart the case studies. Give one to each student group. You may want to mount the case studies on card stock for reuse.

CASE STUDY 1

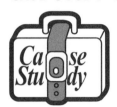

Latasha has just started going out with Franklin, who is 4 years older. She likes kissing and hugging Franklin because it feels really good. Franklin has had lots of other girlfriends and Latasha knows that he had sex with many of them. Franklin has promised Latasha that she will like having sex more than anything else they've done.

CASE STUDY 2

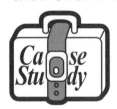

Lee and Jamie have dated for a long time. They decided not to have sex because they believe that sex would change the way they feel about each other and their relationship. Both Lee and Jamie enjoy just spending time together because they enjoy doing so many of the same things. They can talk to each other about *anything*. For a long time, Lee and Jamie's friends have hinted that they are really missing something by not having sex. Jamie doesn't care what their friends say, but Lee thinks they might have a good point. Lee is trying to persuade Jamie to have sex "just once" to see what it's like.

CASE STUDY 3

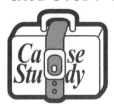

Michael has never had sex because he believes the best way to keep from getting an STD is to remain a virgin. He also thinks it's important to be a positive influence on his little brother and little sisters. Michael knows that his brother and sisters look up to him. He can't tell *them* to abstain from sex if he doesn't practice what he preaches. Michael has been invited to a party where there will be a lot of drinking. Amanda will also be there. Michael and Amanda have done a lot of kissing and touching when they have been together. He is really attracted to Amanda and she has told him that she would like to have sex with him.

MAKING MY CHOICE

Name _____ Date _____ Period _____

 DIRECTIONS Everyone must make a choice about abstinence in his or her life. Situations and circumstances make everyone's choice a personal one. Follow the steps in thinking through the choice of abstinence for yourself.

A. State the problem.

B. List the options.
  1. _____
  2. _____

C. State the consequences.
  Option 1 _____
  1. _____
  2. _____
  3. _____
  4. _____
  5. _____

  Option 2 _____
  1. _____
  2. _____
  3. _____
  4. _____
  5. _____

D. Make the choice.

E. Evaluate the choice.

ABSTINENCE NOW

Name _____ Date _____ Period _____

DIRECTIONS ⟩ What are good reasons to choose to be abstinent during high school?

1.

2.

3.

4.

- **Planning ways to be alone with a partner.**

- **Thinking about touching a partner.**

- **Planning to get and use alcohol or other drugs to relax.**

- **Dressing in a sexy way.**

HANDLING *CAUTION* SITUATIONS

Name _____ Date _____ Period _____

DIRECTIONS ▶ Write down 2 *caution* situations. Then describe how you would handle the situation to follow through on your decision to be abstinent.

EXAMPLE

Caution—You are daydreaming in class about the last time you were with your girlfriend or boyfriend. You really enjoyed kissing and touching and are curious about how it would feel to touch even more.

How to handle the situation—**Decide to invite my best friend to double date the next time we go out, so I can be with my boyfriend or girlfriend without having to be alone.**

Caution #1

How to handle the situation

Caution #2

How to handle the situation

Choosing Health High School

© ETR Associates

- **Touching each other in more ways.**

- **Getting sexually excited.**

- **Removing clothing.**

- **Lying down together.**

1. **Send a nonverbal no (stand tall, firm expression, serious tone of voice).**

2. **Use the word** *no.*

3. **Repeat the no (as often as needed).**

4. **Suggest an alternate activity (something else to do).**

5. **Build the relationship (let other person know you value the relationship).**

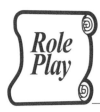

HOW ABOUT A DATE?—
UNCONVINCING VERSION

ROLEPLAY

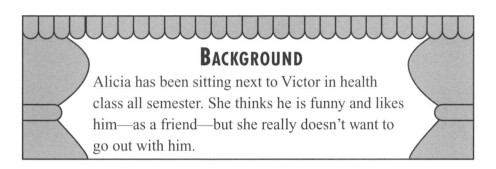

BACKGROUND
Alicia has been sitting next to Victor in health class all semester. She thinks he is funny and likes him—as a friend—but she really doesn't want to go out with him.

Victor: Hey, Alicia, I've decided it's time for us to go out.

Alicia: Well, Victor, you know I'm pretty busy.

Victor: Come on. You know we would have fun.

Alicia: You *are* fun to be around, Victor.

Victor: So, how about this weekend? We could rent a video.

Alicia: I don't know. I may have to babysit my niece.

Victor: Hey, that's OK, you could bring her along.

Alicia: I would have to ask her mom.

Victor: Then I guess it's settled. I'll see you Saturday.

Alicia: I guess I'll see you then.

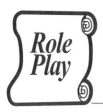 *Role Play*

HOW ABOUT A DATE?—
CONVINCING VERSION

ROLEPLAY

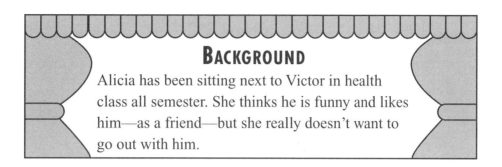

BACKGROUND

Alicia has been sitting next to Victor in health class all semester. She thinks he is funny and likes him—as a friend—but she really doesn't want to go out with him.

Victor: Hey, Alicia, I've decided it's time for us to go out.

Alicia: I'm flattered. But I have to say no.

Victor: Come on. You know we would have fun.

Alicia: We do have fun in class, but I don't want to go out.

Victor: We could rent a video this weekend.

Alicia: No, Victor, I can't. Maybe we could hang out during lunch.

Victor: I guess you just don't like me.

Alicia: You're fun and I really like you, Victor, but just as a friend.

JUST THIS ONCE

Name _____ Date _____ Period _____

DIRECTIONS Complete the dialogue on the script. Use skills to show a convincing refusal.

BACKGROUND

Your friend meets you before school and asks to copy your math homework. It took an hour to work the problems and you really don't feel like letting your friend copy them.

Friend: Boy, am I glad you did your math homework. Let me borrow it until math class.

You:

Friend: Oh, come on. I'd let you copy my homework.

You:

Friend: Let me use your problems just this once. I'll do the math homework tonight and share it with you tomorrow.

You:

Friend: What do you expect me to do if I can't use your problems?

You:

Name _____ Date _____ Period _____

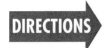 **DIRECTIONS** In Part 1, put a check in front of the statements that use skills for convincing refusals. Then use verbal skills for refusals to write a response for each of the statements in Part 2.

PART 1

_____ a.   I don't think that's a good idea.

_____ b.   No, let's go to the mall.

_____ c.   No. I like to be with you, but I just don't feel comfortable at your house when your parents aren't home.

_____ d.   Probably not. I don't know.

_____ e.   Maybe. I'll think about it.

_____ f.   No, not now. Let's see a movie instead.

PART 2

1. You know you hate Mr. Lubke's class. Let's cut today and have some fun.

2. Your mom won't know if you don't go straight home from school. C'mon, I really need a ride.

Name _____ Date _____ Period _____

DIRECTIONS ▶ Use this checklist to identify the skills for refusals used in the roleplays.

SKILLS	ROLEPLAY		
	Cookies and Yogurt	**Home Alone**	**A Walk in the Park**
Erect posture			
Firm expression			
Serious voice			
Said *no*			
Repeated no			
Suggested an alternate activity			
Built the relationship			

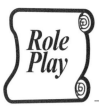
COOKIES AND YOGURT

ROLEPLAY

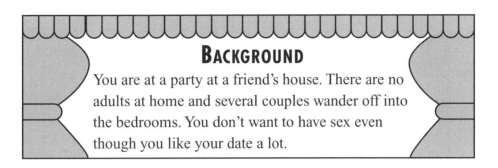

BACKGROUND

You are at a party at a friend's house. There are no adults at home and several couples wander off into the bedrooms. You don't want to have sex even though you like your date a lot.

Date: C'mon, let's go into the bedroom so we can be by ourselves.

You: No, I don't think that's a good idea.

Date: What's the big deal? I'm not asking you to have sex. I just want to get to know you better.

You: I'd like to get to know you better too, but I don't want to be in the bedroom.

Date: I've been looking forward to being alone with you since we met.

You: That's really nice. Why don't we go to my house. My family's there, but we can sit on the porch and talk as long as we want.

Date: I don't think your house will be as private as it is here.

You: It may not be as private, but I can be more relaxed and really get to know you. Besides, we have cookies and frozen yogurt at my house.

Date: OK, you and the cookies have convinced me this time.

You: Great! Let's go.

HOME ALONE

ROLEPLAY

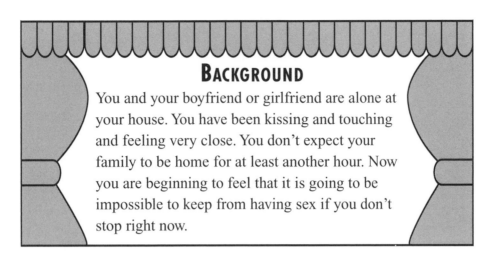

BACKGROUND

You and your boyfriend or girlfriend are alone at your house. You have been kissing and touching and feeling very close. You don't expect your family to be home for at least another hour. Now you are beginning to feel that it is going to be impossible to keep from having sex if you don't stop right now.

You: Wait. If we don't stop now, it's going to be impossible to keep from having sex.

Partner: That's OK. I love you and I don't want to stop this time.

You:

Partner: What's wrong? Don't you love me?

You:

Partner: I don't understand. Nothing bad will happen. We'll just feel closer.

You:

Partner: Don't you care about what I want?

You:

Partner: Sounds like you are really serious. Maybe we need to talk more about our relationship.

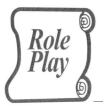

A WALK IN THE PARK

ROLEPLAY

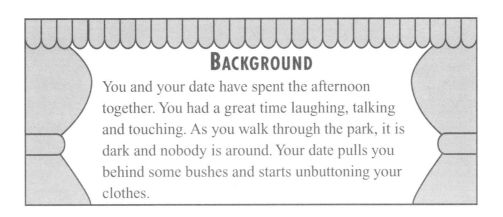

BACKGROUND

You and your date have spent the afternoon together. You had a great time laughing, talking and touching. As you walk through the park, it is dark and nobody is around. Your date pulls you behind some bushes and starts unbuttoning your clothes.

Date: This is great! Let's just let things happen.

You:

Date:

You:

Date:

You:

Date:

You:

You:

Date:

You:

LET'S TALK

Name _____ Date _____ Period _____

DIRECTIONS ➤ Brainstorm topics that a couple may talk about before they have sex. Add the most important topics you have brainstormed to the list below. Then put all the topics in order by writing a "1" beside the topic you feel is easiest to talk about, a "2" by the topic that would be next, etc.

_____ How much they care about each other.

_____ How their relationship will change if they have sex.

_____ Using a condom.

_____ Who will buy the condom.

_____ If they're ready to have sex.

_____ Previous sexual experience.

_____

_____

_____

_____

Choosing Health High School

CONDOM COMMUNICATION

Name _____ Date _____ Period _____

DIRECTIONS ▶ Write what you might say in a conversation with your partner about using condoms.

Partner: You know how much I love you.

You:

Partner: But condoms really spoil the mood, and I would feel stupid buying them.

You:

Partner:

You:

Partner:

You:

Partner:

You:

Choosing Health High School

Name _____ Date _____ Period _____

Discuss using condoms with **P**artner.

Open the package and **R**emove the condom carefully.

Unr**O**ll the condom onto the erect penis, leaving 1/2 inch at the tip.

Add lubrica**T**ion.

Hold the rim of the condom in place when withdrawing the p**E**nis.

Take off the **C**ondom away from partner's genitals.

Throw the used condom away.

PRICING PROTECTION PRODUCTS

Name _____ Date _____ Period _____

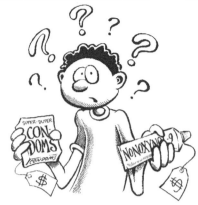

DIRECTIONS 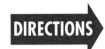 Take this activity sheet to a store where condoms are sold. Collect information about these products to answer the questions.

1. What is the name of the store you visited?

2. In what section of the store were the condoms and/or products containing nonoxynol-9 found?

3. What brands of condoms and nonoxynol-9 products did you find?

4. How much did each of these products cost?

5. How old do you have to be to purchase these products?

6. List 3 feelings you experienced while getting the information about these products.

7. List 3 feelings you think you would experience if you were purchasing one of these products.

STD SYMPTOMS AND CONSEQUENCES

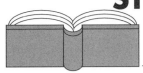

STD	SYMPTOMS	CONSEQUENCES
HIV	Symptoms begin several months to several years after infection. • Flu-like feelings that persist • Unexplained weight loss • Night sweats • Persistent diarrhea • White spots in mouth • Unexplained fatigue	You can give HIV to your sexual partner or someone you share a needle with. HIV cannot be cured. Many people die from it. HIV damages the immune system, making a person susceptible to many different illnesses and infections. Passed from mother to child before, during or after birth (through breastfeeding).
CHLAMYDIA	Symptoms begin 7–21 days after infection. • Most women and some men have no symptoms • Discharge from the sex organs • Burning or pain while urinating • Unusual bleeding from the vagina • Pain in the pelvic area	You can give chlamydia to your sexual partner. Can damage reproductive organs. Can cause sterility. Passed from mother to child during childbirth.
GENITAL WARTS	Symptoms begin 1–6 months after infection. • Small, bumpy warts on and around the sex organs • Itching and burning around the sex organs	You can give genital warts to your sexual partner. More warts can grow. Warts may signal precancerous condition. Passed from mother to child during childbirth.

(continued...)

STD	SYMPTOMS	CONSEQUENCES
GONORRHEA	Symptoms begin 2–21 days after infection. • Most women and some men have no symptoms • Discharge from the sex organs • Burning or pain while urinating or having a bowel movement • Increased pain during menstrual periods • Pain in the pelvic area	You can give gonorrhea to your sexual partner. Can damage reproductive organs. Can cause sterility. Can cause heart trouble, blindness, skin disease, arthritis. Passed from mother to child during childbirth.
HERPES	Symptoms begin 2–30 days after infection. • Flu-like feelings • Small, painful blisters on the sex organs or mouth • Itching and burning around the sex organs before the blisters appear • Blisters last 1-3 weeks • Blisters disappear but the individual still has herpes • Blisters may recur	You can give herpes to your sexual partner. Herpes cannot be cured. Passed from mother to child during childbirth.
SYPHILIS	**1st Stage** Symptoms begin 1–12 weeks after infection. • Painless, open sore on the mouth or sex organ • Sore goes away after 1–5 weeks **2nd Stage** Symptoms begin 1–6 months after sore appears. • A rash anywhere on the body • Flu-like symptoms	You can give syphilis to your sexual partner. Can cause heart disease, brain damage, blindness and death. Passed from mother to fetus during pregnancy.

© ETR Associates

ROSA AND RAMON

CASE STUDY

Name _____ Date _____ Period _____

 DIRECTIONS Read the case study and answer the questions.

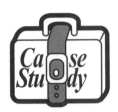 Even though Ramon and Rosa had been attracted to each other for a long time, they just never seemed to get together. When Ramon was available, Rosa was going steady. When Rosa was available, Ramon was seeing someone else. When they finally began to date, Rosa and Ramon fell in love and decided to begin a sexual relationship. Almost a month after Rosa first had intercourse with Ramon, she developed a fever and headache. Small fluid-filled blisters appeared on her sex organs.

1. Which STD might Rosa have?

2. How can Rosa be cured?

3. What might happen if Rosa becomes pregnant?

MELISSA AND JOSH

CASE STUDY

Name _____ Date _____ Period _____

DIRECTIONS ▶ Read the case study and answer the questions.

Melissa and Josh met at college and dated during their senior year. They made plans to marry after graduation. Two weeks before the wedding, Josh told Melissa that he has genital warts.

1. What symptoms probably alerted Josh to his condition?

2. What might happen if Melissa and Josh have unprotected intercourse?

3. Could Melissa get genital warts if Josh uses a condom and she uses nonoxynol-9?

4. What are the consequences of genital warts?

CASE STUDY

Name _____ Date _____ Period _____

DIRECTIONS ▶ Read the case study and answer the questions.

Frederick was proud to join the U.S. Navy after high school graduation. While in basic training, he began to visit a local pool hall on weekends. One night, Frederick went home with someone he had just met at the pool hall. Several weeks after this 1-night stand, Frederick noticed a sore on his penis. He was concerned at first, but the sore didn't hurt and it disappeared after a couple of weeks.

1. Which STD does Frederick probably have?

2. Since his symptoms went away, is he cured?

3. What will the next symptoms probably be?

4. What will happen if Frederick does not get treated?

MICHAEL AND SUNNY

CASE STUDY

Name _____ Date _____ Period _____

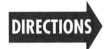 **DIRECTIONS** Read the case study and answer the questions.

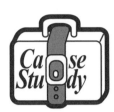 Sunny and Michael were filled with joy when they discovered Sunny was pregnant. Not long after this exciting news, Michael realized that something was wrong. He developed diarrhea, had no appetite and lost a lot of weight. Michael often felt tired even when he was getting enough sleep.

1. Which STD might Michael have?

2. How could Michael have gotten this STD?

3. What are the consequences of this STD for Michael, Sunny and their unborn child?

Name _____ Date _____ Period _____

Complete the items that are assigned to your group.

Group member names:

1. Think of a question about STD that has not been answered in class. Write it here.

2. The STD hotline number:

3. Call the number and ask your question. Write the answer here.

4. Think of a question about HIV infection. Write it here.

5. The HIV hotline number:

(continued…)

CONTINUED

6. Call the number and ask your question. Write the answer here.

7. How did you feel when you called the hotline?

8. Was the person who answered your questions helpful? courteous? easily understood? Explain.

9. Locally, where could you receive STD information, a test, checkup or treatment?

   Clinic Name:

   Address:

   Phone:

   Office hours:

   Cost:

   Is a visit to the clinic confidential?   Yes   No

STD SLEUTH CLUES

DIRECTIONS Cut apart the clue strips and distribute them among 5 separate envelopes. Make sure that each envelope contains no more than 2 clues for the same STD.

HIV Infection

It's the immune system's worst enemy.

Sweating at night is a cause of fright.

May take several months to show up on a blood test.

Breastfeeding may be hazardous.

Chlamydia or Gonorrhea

A woman may not know she has it.

Discharge is an unwelcome sign.

A trip to the restroom is unforgettable.

A delay in treatment may mean no babies ever.

Genital Warts

Small and bumpy signs of trouble.

Increased risk for cancer is always there.

Burn them or freeze them but they may come back.

Caused by a virus, not by frogs.

(continued...)

Choosing Health High School

STD Sleuth Clues

CONTINUED

Herpes

| May think it's the flu until blisters arrive. |
| When under stress, symptoms may come back. |
| Feel better in 1–3 weeks. |
| The mouth and genitals are usual places. |

Syphilis

| Stages are not just for theaters. |
| A rash can appear most anywhere. |
| After a while, the heart and brain know. |
| The sore doesn't hurt, but the disease can kill. |

DR. KNOW

Name _____ Date _____ Period _____

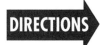 **DIRECTIONS** Read the letter. Then answer the questions as you learn more about HIV.

Dear Dr. Know,

    I never thought I would be writing to you for advice, but here I go. I have heard a lot about HIV and AIDS on TV and have read about them in the newspaper. Is HIV infection the same as AIDS? It seems that everything I read and hear is scary and confusing.

    Sometimes I wonder if *everyone* will end up getting this disease! I will be graduating from high school before too long and want to have a happy and *long* life. What causes HIV, and how do people get it? What are the symptoms? How can I keep from getting HIV? How can I tell if I have it? These may seem like dumb questions to you, but knowing the answers would make my life easier.

                Signed,
                16 and Needing Answers

---

1. Is HIV infection the same as AIDS?

2. What causes HIV infection?

3. How do people get HIV?

(continued...)

DR. KNOW

CONTINUED

4. What are the symptoms of HIV infection?

5. How can I tell if I have HIV?

6. How can I protect myself from HIV?